THE
CONQUEST
OF
CANCER

THE CONQUEST OF Cancer

VACCINES AND DIET

**Virginia Livingston-Wheeler, M.D.
and Edmond G. Addeo**

With an Introduction by
ALSOPH H. CORWIN, Ph.D., D.Sc. (Hon)
Professor of Chemistry, Emeritus,
Johns Hopkins University

FRANKLIN WATTS
New York London Toronto Sydney 1984

The material contained in this book is not meant
to be a manual for self-treatment, nor should it
be a substitute for the advice of a physician.

Library of Congress Cataloging in Publication Data

Livingston-Wheeler, Virginia.
The conquest of cancer.

Bibliography: p.
Includes index.
1. Cancer—Prevention. 2. Cancer—Preventive
inoculation. 3. Cancer—Diet therapy. I. Addeo,
Edmond G., 1936–   . II. Title.
RC268.L58 1983   616.99'406   83-14502
ISBN 0-531-09806-0

TABLE OF CONTENTS

This book is gratefully dedicated to my loving
and helpful collaborator, partner and husband,
Dr. Owen Webster Wheeler,
and to the patients of the Livingston-Wheeler Clinic.

INTRO-DUCTION

ALSOPH H. CORWIN,
Ph.D., D. Sc. (Hon), Professor
of Chemistry, Emeritus
Johns Hopkins University

IN CERTAIN QUARTERS the cause of cancer is still highly controversial. Some virologists maintain that cancer is the manifestation of a viral infection. Many oncologists believe that most cancers consist of lumps formed by the uncontrolled growth of cells that have been caused to mutate by chemicals or radiation. There may be a germ of truth in each point of view. Dr. Virginia Livingston-Wheeler and her collaborators have studied the cancer problem in the laboratory and in the clinic for four decades. Their numerous published scientific papers demonstrate that the full explanation lies in a third direction, namely, that cancers are caused by a microbial infective agent, as shown by Dr. Peyton Rous in 1910. This agent can exist in a filterable form, which makes it appear to some that it is a virus. The organism also has the power of performing a feat of genetic engineering by hybridizing with host cells, conferring upon them invasive and toxic properties. Until the relatively recent discoveries in genetics, such a change could have been explained most logically as caused by mutation brought on from an outside source. As a result of Dr. Virginia's publications, which have been confirmed by numerous independent scientists around the world, the remarkable powers of the cancer organism can now be understood.

Building logically upon the information that cancer is a generalized infection, not a localized phenomenon, the Livingston-Wheeler approach has achieved valuable clinical results which are presented in this volume. Physicians who are not acquainted with her earlier compendium *The Microbiology of Cancer* would be well advised to study it, along with the pertinent subsequent scientific publications. These earlier works form the backdrop to the present volume, which is intended for the lay public as well as for those in the medical profession who may not have become acquainted with this overwhelmingly important field. Lay readers will find in it food for thought and encouragement in their quest for better health.

COLLAB-ORATOR'S NOTE

In January of 1980, at an Orthomolecular Medical Society meeting in San Francisco, I listened to Dr. Virginia Livingston-Wheeler present a paper on the immunotherapy program of the Livingston-Wheeler Medical Clinic in San Diego.

Dr. Virginia (as she is called by friends and colleagues), with the aid of her husband, Dr. Owen Webster Wheeler, presented a wealth of scientific data as she explained her discovery of the cancer-causing microbe *Progenitor Cryptocides* and her successful treatment program that emphasizes the strengthening of patients' immune systems. She described a treatment program that consists of giving patients (1) antitubercular vaccines (BCG) to boost immune response, (2) autogenous vaccines prepared from a culture of each patient's own *Progenitor Cryptocides* microbes, (3) high doses of vitamins such as A, C, E and essential minerals, and (4) a special immunity-boosting diet which promotes general health while avoiding cancer-promoting foods.

Dr. Virginia concluded her speech by reporting that, although her treatment program could still be expanded, she was achieving an improvement rate among her patients in excess of 90 percent.

The austere medical audience gave her a ten minute standing ovation.

I spent the next two years becoming more familiar with orthomolecular medicine in general and the work of Dr. Livingston-Wheeler in particular. I learned that Dr. Livingston-Wheeler had more than forty years experience in medicine and that while a Professor of Microbiology at Rutgers University and the University of San Diego her work had been applauded at major scientific meetings from Rome to Paris to New York; that her scientific papers and articles had appeared in prominent scientific journals; and that she was listed in several *Who's Who* of science and medicine.

In June of 1982, I was fortunate enough to meet William Gladstone, president of Waterside Productions, a literary agency based in Del Mar, California. Mr. Gladstone is a good friend of Dr. Livingston-Wheeler's and was looking for a seasoned medical writer to help bring her message to the American public. With three medical books to my credit along with seven others, I was given the opportunity to collaborate on the writing of this book.

I soon found myself engrossed in what I now consider to be one of the most exciting and significant medical breakthroughs of the twentieth century. After many hours of conversation with Dr. Virginia and her husband and colleague, Dr. Owen Wheeler, after extensive interviews with her patients, days spent at the clinic, and reviews of hundreds of their patients' medical charts, I am convinced that Dr. Virginia's work is as important as the work of Louis Pasteur, Madame Curie, or Salk and Sabin.

If you are reading this book because you have cancer, you are about to discover a treatment program that puts the odds of surviving to live a healthy, comfortable, productive life in your favor. If you do not have cancer, you are about to discover a program that will diminish the likelihood that you will ever suffer from this dreaded disease. Along the way you will learn the compelling story of Dr. Virginia's lifetime of medical research to find a cure for this treacherous disease.

Edmond G. Addeo
Mill Valley, Calif.

1
WHY NOW?

BILLIONS OF DOLLARS have been misspent over the years in the attempt to prevent or cure cancer. Despite these billions of dollars and the fact that the possibility for cure has existed for decades, cancer is on the increase. Why? It has been known for more than fifty years that cancer is an infectious disease. A mysterious virus has been sought in sophisticated research laboratories across the country, yet still hasn't been found.

These are strong statements. I intend, with this book, to show that they are true. After years of neglect by the cancer establishment, I have decided to bring my case for the conquest of cancer to the American public. There *is* a vaccine against cancer and it is available to anyone.

Early in this century, Dr. Peyton Rous demonstrated that 90 percent of the chickens for sale in New York City were cancerous. He defined the poultry infection as caused by an unknown microbial agent that passed through a special filter designed to hold back bacteria but not viruses. The filtrability of this "cancer agent" led to the erroneous belief that a virus was responsible for cancer, but my research has confirmed that this is not true.

Various discoveries made over the course of my career have led to the conclusion that cancer is caused by a bacterium, which I have formally classified as *Progenitor Cryptocides*. Moreover, this bacterium can be isolated and cultured, and a vaccine can be made from it that can help your immune system keep cancer suppressed and, if it appears, can help fight it off. This disease is definitely transmissible to man from animals, and because the cancer-causing microbe also already exists in our bodies from birth, it is immuno-therapy that is the single most powerful anti-cancer program for all kinds of cancers. I predict that in ten years immunotherapy will be the prevailing treatment of cancer patients.

This book is the story of my discoveries and how they are being applied today to help patients recover through immunotherapy.

It all started in 1947 when I was a school doctor in Newark, New Jersey. I had been graduated from New York University–Bellevue Medical College as one of four women doctors in my class and had served as the first woman resident in New York City, in the infectious disease section of a hospital prison ward. During the war I worked as an industrial physician at Western Electric, and when the war ended I went to work at various medical jobs. After a long wait my husband and I adopted a baby, and when we moved to Newark I took the school job to help make ends meet. Jobs were scarce.

As with most important discoveries, it seems, it was quite by accident that I discovered the positive identification of the microorganism that causes cancer. A school nurse had asked me to look at a worrisome condition she had, a disease that greatly resembled leprosy. In the infectious disease ward of the hospital in Brooklyn where I had interned, I had seen many different kinds of infectious diseases, among them leprosy, and I had taken a keen research interest in this field. This woman had ulcers on her fingers, hardening of the skin, and a perforation in her nasal septum. She had no sensation of hot or cold on the affected areas. These symptoms are characteristic of leprosy, but her own doctor had diagnosed her condition as scleroderma, which is a hardening and rigid thickening of the skin.

The nurse didn't have leprosy, but out of sheer curiosity I made some smears of the nasal lesion and of the ulcers on her fingers. I stained them with Ziehl-Neelsen stain, which is customarily used to identify leprosy and tuberculosis. To my astonishment I saw under the microscope the same kind of microorganisms that are seen in leprosy. The microbes were red-staining, or "acid-fast." Although the nurse didn't have leprosy, I had found in her an acid-fast microorganism that was neither the lepra bacillus nor the tubercle bacillus. At the time, I called it sclerobacillus and reasoned that it must be the causative agent in scleroderma and possibly other diseases. I then treated the nurse with some medications that are used in treating leprosy. To my gratification her lesions began to heal.

When I began to treat other patients with scleroderma and Raynaud's syndrome the same way, they, too, healed. My curiosity was further aroused. So I set up a research laboratory in our basement at home where I studied this strange microorganism that I had discovered to be acid-fast and pleomorphic (assuming many different shapes) but definitely not the lepra or tubercle bacillus.

Subsequently, I met Dr. Eleanor Alexander-Jackson, who was doing significant work with tuberculosis, and who was studying the pleomorphic forms of that particular microbe. I started to visit her regularly at her laboratory at Cornell University, and we worked together closely on pleomorphism in scleroderma and other collagen diseases such as lupus erythematosis and erythema nodosum. (These collagen diseases cause a conspicuous alteration in connective tissues, in which the malformation of cells is involved.)

I will relate the details of this exciting period in my life in a later chapter, but for now the critical thing is that I found that *when I inoculated animals with this acid-fast microbe, many of them developed cancer.* I thought this was extremely unusual and decided to find out more about cancer. Through numerous medical contacts I was able to obtain small pieces of tumors and make literally thousands of slides from them. I was astounded to find that when I applied the Ziehl-Neelsen stain, the identical appearing microbes were present in all cancers.

I decided then to go directly into the operating rooms and get tissues that had no possibility of contamination. I haunted the local hospitals in New Jersey and New York City and stained tissue after tissue. I used the most rigid techniques for sterility and yet time and again found the same microbe in every single slide I prepared. Moreover, when I cultured this microbe from tissues and patients' blood and injected it into mice, *many mice developed cancer* or a related collagen disease.

I was almost speechless with amazement. I knew that a number of scientists had claimed that cancer was caused by a microbe—Doyen in France, Mori in Italy, and many others—but they didn't know it was acid-fast and were told by their peers that it was just a contaminant and didn't signify anything important. I was just a lowly school doctor who now wanted to proclaim to the medical world that cancer was caused by a microbe, an acid-fast bacillus, and I could demonstrate it. I published a few papers in local professional journals, such as the *New Jersey State Medical Journal*, but couldn't get the attention of the major periodicals.

However, I eventually affiliated with Rutgers University and received many grants to pursue my research into the cause and cure of cancer. These events are related in detail later.

That was about forty years ago. I have decided that this story, and the story of the remarkable success rate we are having at our clinic in San Diego, must now be told to the American public. The immunotherapy treatments we have employed to help in the recovery of many hundreds of cancer victims are the result of almost half a century of extensive research *and* clinical practice and are now ready to be made available to as wide a public as possible.

Because the microbe I independently discovered to be acid-fast and etiologically related to cancer is a bacterium, and not a virus as conventional medicine insists, and because I involve *diet* heavily in the immunotherapy program we have developed, the conventional body of the American Medical Society and the American Cancer Society have not yet recognized our work at the clinic. However, we are working in close cooperation with dozens of local surgeons and specialists in the cancer community, and hundreds of physicians in America and abroad have sent their patients to us and seen them return home on the road to recovery. It is because of these wonderful results that I have decided to publish the whole story.

If current trends continue, you or someone you love will be stricken with cancer within the next ten years. The chances are as much as one in four that you yourself will contract cancer. If you are over sixty years of age, the chances are one in three. Because cancer is usually without pain or other symptoms in its early stages, there is a chance you have it right now and do not know it.

Despite technological advancements in surgery, radiation, and chemotherapy—the three "approved" cancer treatments— your chances of avoiding cancer have not been improving. Americans continue to smoke cigarettes, embrace nutritionally bankrupt diets, drink fluoridated water, breathe polluted air, and contaminate the surf we swim in, the bays and seas that give us our fish, and even the land on which we grow our food with hundreds of environmental pollutants. In fact, those three traditional therapeutic treatments for cancer, in many cases, may even *shorten* your life. The obvious reality is that they do nothing to help you prevent the disease from striking in the first place.

Breakthroughs in the past ten years have pointed the way to a biological cure for cancer, one based on preventing the onset of the disease from the beginning. The keystone of these breakthroughs has been enhancing the individual's immune system with proper diet and vaccines. My research for the causes of cancer led me to believe in the "strong diet = strong immunity" concept of disease prevention. For the last fourteen years I have been achieving remarkable results with human cancer patients by using immunotherapy techniques to help their own bodies ward off the tumors and literally destroy them. These immuno-therapy techniques include the formulation of an autogenous vaccine (i.e., a vaccine made from specific microbes in the patient's own body fluids or tumors), a strict high immunity diet, and high doses of certain important anti-cancer vitamins (such as vitamins A, C and E) as well as other nutrients. This entire concept is immeasurably strengthened by the fact that *Progenitor Cryptocides* produces choriogonadotropins (CG), an essential hormone, in the test tube. I made this discovery in 1970, and it is now confirmed worldwide. In 1977 the fact that a microbe produces CG in nature led to the approval of genetic engineering by the government.

Therefore, while much in this book will seem new to you, it has already stood the test of time—in some cases twenty-five or thirty years of continuous experimentation—which even in the most conservative of circles should be enough evidence to begin investigating the results.

No matter what stage of cancer you or a loved one has, immediate implementation of the Livingston Anti-Cancer Diet can help strengthen your immune system and fortify you in the battle against your disease. Change in diet alone may not cure you. But it can make a vital difference in the course of the cancer. More importantly, for those of you who have not yet been stricken, a variation of the diet which we call the Livingston Cancer Prevention Diet can be a strong safeguard against coming down with this dread disease.

You will not find our clinic in San Diego or our immuno-therapy methods on the approved list of the American Cancer Society. This is because, nutritionally speaking, traditional medicine is only now stepping out of the Middle Ages. Let us not forget that it took almost 250 years to convince surgeons to wash their hands before entering the operating room.

People continue to die of cancer, yet the techniques we have developed at our clinic have enabled many so-called terminal cancer patients to reverse their diseases and even live out the rest of their lives free of tumors and pain. Many respected physicians, surgeons, and university scientists have visited the clinic and been impressed with the results. Many others are duplicating our work at their own hospital laboratories and university research centers. Several great institutions, such as Duke University, have invited us to present seminars on our work. However, the A.M.A. and the American Cancer Society officially have not recognized us, even though we *do*, in fact, employ the conventional modalities of radiation, surgery, and chemotherapy when they are indicated, but *only* when indicated and not as a matter of routine. Further, radiation and chemotherapy are used *only* in carefully controlled doses.

It is astounding to me that a "respected" group of scientists and physicians on the National Research Council of the National Academy of Sciences published in June 1982 a National Cancer Institute-sponsored report (*Diet, Nutrition and Cancer*, National Academy Press) on the relationship between diet and cancer and simply asked Americans to eat more food containing vitamins A and C. Not once did the report suggest vitamin supplements or that perhaps the food the typical American eats *does not have* the high level of nutrition it is supposed to have. The report suggested "a reduction" of the intake of red meat, but it didn't report that a large number of slaughtered cattle are infected with cancer. Nor did the report mention the percentage of commercial chickens which have visible cancer when slaughtered.

I believe an alarmingly high percentage of commercial chickens, in the range of nine out of ten, have the *pathogenic* form of the cancer microbe, and it is transmissable from the hen to the egg to the chick. Chapter Nine will examine this further, but for now the point is that the very idea of avoiding some foods totally and eating more of other foods to prevent and even cure cancer is anathema to the American medical establishment. This overall attitude toward new ideas and the reluctance to accept clinical results as a stimulus for further investigation is not much different from the attitude under which Louis Pasteur was hooted off the stage at the Academy of Sciences in Paris for suggesting that milk be boiled before it was given to children because it had infectious "microbes" in it.

The biological approach to cancer prevention and treatment should be, but is not, accepted by those who specialize in radiation and chemical treatment, as an enhancement and detoxification of the side effects of their own methods. I honestly don't know *why* these practitioners don't accept it—perhaps it has something to do with the vested interests of the medical establishment. Others contend it's merely the result of inertia and the outmoded approach to medical instruction that is still predominant in medical schools. Or, perhaps, it is because in modern America technological methods receive the most attention in scientific journals and government funding.

I must also state here that I fully expect controversial reaction to our program and that, indeed, I have grown accustomed to it. I graduated from medical school when there was severe discrimination against women in the medical profession. Ever since then, controversy has followed my work.

The microbe I discovered to be acid-fast and classified as *Progenitor Cryptocides* is a bacillus that is a first cousin to the bacilli that cause tuberculosis and leprosy. I believed then, and have proven repeatedly, that this P. *Cryptocides* bacillus is the causative agent of cancer—all cancers. This microbe is present in all of our cells, and it is only our immune systems that keep it suppressed. When our immune systems are weakened, either by poor diet, infected foods, or old age, this microbe gains a foothold and starts cancer cells growing into tumors. This immune system principle is the entire basis for our program in San Diego. The microbe is an obligate symbiant, meaning that it is contained within the normal cell in symbiosis, emerges after injury during the healing process, but when not immunologically and nutritionally controlled it produces neoplastic cells. It is a function of the normal cell but reverts to a pathogenic state, a bacterial revertant, when uncontrolled.

Although the experiments in our laboratories and our clinical successes have repeatedly demonstrated the importance of good nutrition in preventing and treating cancer through immunotherapy, only recently has this concept begun to be accepted in the medical community. (I say "begun" because many competent physicians today are using nutrition in their treatments but are still considered "out of the mainstream.") While I know the information in this book will be repeated in the years to come as younger researchers duplicate our work, the traditional medical community is only in the early stages of exploration. In essence, I have a forty-year headstart on them, and the benefits of my research are here for you to put into practice today.

Such "new findings" showing that good nutrition is essential for immunity to cancer will, I'm sure, continue to appear. After all, the connection between what you eat and your level of resistance to cancer and other diseases has already been established, especially by Dr. Linus Pauling and several others (*Cancer and Vitamin C*, by Pauling and Dr. Ewan Cameron).

Our research is still in progress, and we are discovering new things every year. Our treatment program is such that it can be modified each time new information has been tested and verified. None of our treatments harm the body, as radiation and chemotherapy do. The diet program we recommend, although capable of being improved, is the most advanced nutritional approach to immunotherapy available today. The autogenous vaccine we have developed appears to immunize our patients against the very disease that brought them to our doors. When necessary, we do combine our biological approach with surgery, radiation, and chemotherapy. We prefer that our patients avoid these treatments before they come to us, but often they come to us after having been so heavily treated that their immune systems are all but destroyed, and their tumors are far advanced. Indeed, some of the patients have come into the clinic barely able to walk and yet have returned home only weeks later on the road to recovery.

I do not claim to have all the answers, nor do I have a corner on the science of immunotherapy. But we at the clinic have dedicated our lives to helping others, and we continue to treat patients with all stages of cancer. We realize, though, that we can help even more by sharing our findings with others throughout the world. That is why our doors are open to everyone; our facilities and laboratories may be visited by any qualified researcher, oncologist, or scientific organization.

We have tried to present this book in a highly communicative fashion, with the scientific principles involved easily understandable to the lay reader. I have chosen a professional writer with knowledge of medical science as a collaborator. While some technical terms are unavoidable in discussing cancer and its causes, we have tried to simplify the terminology as much as possible. When appropriate, we will define words and concepts parenthetically throughout the narrative. We've also included a glossary of important terms and phrases. I encourage you to refer to it frequently.

After reading this, I hope you will understand one thing: Having cancer doesn't mean you are automatically going to die of it. I hope you will understand the essentials of our biological approach to combating and controlling this frightful disease. Follow the guidelines of our cancer prevention diet, and you will greatly diminish your own chances of getting cancer. To those who already have it, I can only promise you that hundreds have already discovered that their tumors have diminished or disappeared completely after they embraced our immunotherapy program and anti-cancer diet.

Since cancer appears to be an immune deficiency disease based on definite inadequacies of such nutrients as the retinoic acids, on specific components of vitamin A as well as on many other complex dietary factors, no other treatment program today offers so much hope and promise in preventing and curing cancer.

2

100
RANDOM
CASE
HISTORIES

WHEN I GIVE A LECTURE to a professional group I am frequently asked for statistics regarding the success rate at our clinic. My reply up to now has been that we have been too experimentally involved in an ongoing program to offer an overall statistical study of our patients adequate for public release. There is also the problem of quantifying many different conditions for comparison with each other. For example, how does one compare a rectal tumor that has metastasized to the liver with a single small node in the breast requiring a simple mastectomy? Suppose the latter patient adopts our program and becomes completely clear with no recurrence, whereas the former patient has his tumor removed and while on the program finds that his liver lesion has disappeared but then drops the program and has a recurrence? How do we compare the two cases? Two remissions? One remission and one failure?

In any event, a formal statistical analysis is currently being attempted with the help of a new computer system installed at the clinic. Meanwhile, we thought it would be useful to present a random survey of 100 patients from the charts in our files. These were our ground rules:

- All of our patients have had their specific diagnoses made by qualified pathologists before coming to us.
- Someone not employed by our clinic drew 100 charts from our files, totally at random and without examining either the name of the patient or the type of condition involved.
- When we examined a chart and found that the patient was *not* a cancer patient—i.e., had come to the clinic for hepatitis or allergies or some affliction other than cancer—we excluded the chart.
- In cases where the patient had left the clinic and returned home and had not contacted the clinic in more than a year, we telephoned the patient for a report. We have indicated such telephone follow-ups in the study.
- Many patients come to the clinic against the wishes of their physicians. When they leave the clinic some of these patients are dissuaded by their physicians from continuing the program and then stop taking their vaccines and go off their immunity diets. They then continue with their own physicians' recommendations—radiation, chemotherapy, or whatever. We have excluded these cases, too, from the study.
- We also excluded patients who "went home to die," i.e., were too weak and ill to carry out the program. The study includes only those patients who continued with the program after leaving the clinic or whose conditions were so dramatically improved *at the time they went off the program* that their cases nevertheless warrant examination.
- We have excluded patients who had only recently checked into the clinic, or whose cases were so recent that even the dramatically fast reversals could only be labeled inconclusive. For this reason, patients who first came to the clinic *after* June 30, 1982, were excluded.
- The temptation was great to exclude *all* 1982 patients. However, it is the nature of random selection that some cases will be more recent than others. The reader may wonder about the present status of patients who visited us in the first half 1982, that is, whether it is too soon to declare them recovered.

However, I maintain that if a patient visits us and is on the road to recovery even within *three weeks*, and upon confirmation several months later is still in good health, then that is certainly better than the patient would be if they hadn't come to us at all. Moreover, we are developing new treatments which appear to be much more effective than our previous versions; hence the early 1982 patients *are more likely* to be benefiting more rapidly from our immunotherapy than any of our patients since the clinic began. So, to preserve scientific integrity in this random sampling, if a patient with a tumor visited us as recently as early 1982, then we must report the condition of that patient at the time of this writing, one year later.

■ We were left with 62 charts, and this is the number on which our percentage calculations are based (we have rounded off fractions).

■ In many cases, the patient's condition is much more complicated than described. We have simplified it in order to convey the essence of the problem to the layman. More technical descriptions would be suitable only for a medical doctor.

■ Especially interesting cases that we could not intentionally include in a random sampling are presented in an appendix at the end of this book. As the title of the Appendix indicates, I offer these cases more to the medical profession than to the layman.

These are the totals of the study:
Seventeen of the 62 cases were officially diagnosed as terminal. Four cases died or are presumed dead. The types of cancer broke down as follows:

8 breast and nodes
5 breast
4 breast and lungs
3 breast and rib

1 breast and uterine
2 lung and liver
2 lung and nodes
1 lung and neck, oat-cell
1 uterine
2 uterine and liver
1 uterine and rectal
1 ovaries and uterus
1 ovaries and colon
1 ovaries and nodes
3 colon and liver
3 colon
6 melanomas
2 skin basal cell
3 prostate
1 kidney and liver
1 kidney
1 pancreatic and liver
1 pelvic
1 esophagus
1 larynx
6 Hodgkin's disease

An examination of the 62 random cases shows that our success rate has been 82 percent. Considering the patients we called inconclusive but for whom we were able to be of *some* help, it is over 90 percent.

Now compare our figures with the official (as of early 1983) American Cancer Society figure of 15 percent of patients who are helped by radiation or chemotherapy. (Also, note that the two physicians in our sampling elected not to be treated with radiation or chemotherapy. We find this to be true of practically all the physician-patients who come to our clinic.)

Of the people we could not help, those who died or are presumed dead, I am willing to state that we probably could have helped these patients had they not come to us with enormously debilitated immune systems resulting from having already under-gone massive chemotherapy or radiation. The profound sadness we at the clinic experience when we receive a patient who already is beyond help is only offset by the great joy and satisfaction we feel when so-called terminal patients walk out of our doors after the accepted tests show them to be on the road to recovery, or when the disease is at least controlled to the point where they are able to lead comfortable and normal lives.

Each patient cited here has been proved to have cancer by a qualified pathologist examining tissue under a microscope. In medicine only this represents the final proof of cancer. Once the diagnosis is firmly established, the metastases or recurrences may be judged by other means, such as X ray, CAT scan, and palpating (feeling) nodules. Since people who do not work in the cancer field may not be familiar with some of the terms we use, brief definitions follow.

1. Cancer. A disease in which certain body cells multiply un-controllably and destroy the cells around them. The tech-nical terms for specific cancers are derived from the type of cells which change to become cancer cells.
2. Carcinoma. A malignant new growth derived from epithelial cells tending to infiltrate the surrounding tissues and give rise to metastasis.
3. Melanoma. A malignant tumor formed by the cells in the skin layer which make small granules containing the coloring substance, melanin. It is these cells which become active to give us a suntan. The malignant potential, or killing ability, of melanomas varies greatly, so a system of grading them is uniformly used. As the melanoma gains in malignant po-tential it grows into the skin. Therefore, a Level I melanoma, which is on the surface, is least lethal. A Level II is slightly deeper and more dangerous; a Level III goes through the skin and is much worse; and a Level IV enters the tissue beneath the skin and is worst of all. By knowing these levels for each patient with melanoma, you will have a better idea

of the killing potential of the melanoma and therefore a better appreciation of the effectiveness of the treatment.

4.   Breast Cancers. Cancers that usually develop from the milk glands in the breast and are called adenocarcinomas. The presence of positive lymph nodes and whether the patient is premenopausal or postmenopausal are factors in the approach to treatment.

5.   Hodgkin's Disease. A cancerous transformation of cells in the lymph nodes. There is a complex system of treatments set out for this disease, and some real progress is being made with the standard anti-cancer methods. Hodgkin's disease does tend to get better with time or go into remission, and its capricious course has caused many physicians to be fooled into believing they have cured it.

6.   Sarcoma. A cancer of connective tissues of the body, such as bones, tendons, muscles, bladder, kidney, liver, or lungs. These cancers are as deadly as the carcinomas and usually grow in the same way. In general, these cancers have not responded as well to the usual anti-cancer therapies.

7.   Ovarian Cancer. A cancer that can spread from the ovaries to the peritoneal cavity or belly. Some progress is being made with this disease with standard therapy.

8.   Prostate Cancer. A cancer that ranges in malignant potential from mild to lethal within six months of diagnosis. This cancer may respond to early surgery (removal of the prostate), radiation and estrogen therapy temporarily. In evaluating our treatment we keep this very much in mind and only feel sure we have helped if the cancer has spread into bones or lungs and then regressed. When it has gone this far and responds to our immunotherapy, it is safe to say that we have reversed its course.

9.   Leukemia. A general term for cancer of the white blood cells. There are several types of white blood cells, and their usual function is to fight off infection. The type of leukemia is named for the particular white blood cell that becomes

cancerous. Lymphatic leukemia, for instance, is a cancer of the lymphocytes while myelogenous leukemia involves the polyniorphonuclear cells. Acute leukemia usually requires chemotherapy and marrow transplant as the immune blood cells are not functional. Chronic lymphocytic leukemia may exist for years and may be improved by immunotherapy. Chronic myelogenous leukemia is less responsive to all treatments but may be impaired by immunotherapy.

To avoid tedious repetition we have used certain phrases in our descriptions:

- *the standard program of immunotherapy, usual program,* or *our immunotherapy* refers to the treatment regimen described in Chapter Ten. It includes the use of autogenous and other vaccines to boost immunity, a diet excluding carcinogens and the patient's allergens, nutritional therapy, whole fresh blood transfusions as indicated, and antibodies for treating infections. The diet includes immunity-boosting ingredients such as vitamin A and its derivatives retinoic acid such as the abscissins.
- *at the time of this writing* means October 20, 1983.
- *clear* means having no evidence of cancer detectable by the accepted testing methods, such as ultrasound, body scans, blood chemistry, and X-ray, as well as physical examination and indicated laboratory tests.

So here they are. The randomly selected cases are presented here in no particular order, with no identification to ensure the privacy of the patient. They represent patients from various parts of the United States and foreign countries.

1. —— *A fifty-three-year-old female who came to the clinic in January 1978 with cancer of the right breast and metastasis to the spine and hip. A previous mastectomy had been done ten years*

earlier on the left breast, and a pin had been placed in her leg after it had broken from metastasis. She had undergone several courses of chemotherapy but had decided to stop when lesions continued to grow. We placed her on a standard program of immunotherapy. In January of 1983, a bone scan showed she was completely clear. A telephone check at the time of this writing indicated she had returned to work and felt well.

2. —— *A fifty-six-year-old female who came to the clinic in January 1981 with recurrent intraductal cancer of the right breast. She had had a left mastectomy in 1980, with six positive nodes and a thyroid nodule removed. Follow-up chemotherapy had not prevented a recurrence of another malignant lymph node, and the patient elected to come to the clinic rather than have a second surgery. We placed her on the standard program of immunotherapy. Echograms at the end of 1982 showed she was clear of cancer. A bone scan was also negative in 1982, and a recent visit at the time of this writing showed her still clear.*

3. —— *A forty-year-old male who came to the clinic in November 1981, from the Mayo Clinic. His pathology report indicated nodular sclerosing Hodgkin's disease. He received the standard program of immunotherapy and then had the nodules removed by surgery while staying on his immune program. After immunotherapy he had a further precautionary course of radiation, a laporatomy, and a splenectomy, at which time he was told he was free of disease. A radiology report at the time of this writing indicated that he is clear of cancer and leading a normal life.*

4. —— *A fifty-nine-year-old female who came to the clinic in September 1976. A pathology report at the time of a right radical mastectomy in February 1976 indicated intraductal cancer. She had no previous radiation or chemotherapy. She received our usual program in addition to having several small, left supraclavicular nodes excised. She has remained cancer-free on the preventive program at the time of this writing.*

5. —— A *fifty-nine-year-old female who came to the clinic in October 1973 with a pathology report of basal cell carcinoma of the lip and low-grade cancer of the thyroglossal duct. She had a pelvic complaint. Since cancer is multi-local, she had dilatation and curettage (D & C) of the uterus which detected severe hyperplasia of the lining of the uterus. She was put on the usual program with additional preventive vaccines. A telephone check at the time of this writing indicated she is still clear of cancer and feeling well after local followup.*

6. —— A *fifty-two-year-old female who came to the clinic in March 1981 with a history of cancer of the left breast and metastatic cancer of the lung. She had had a radical mastectomy and radiation for recurrent disease, confirmed by pathology as infiltrating ductal adenocarcinoma. Her diagnosis was labeled "advanced terminal." At the time she responded well to immunotherapy. A chest examination in January 1983 indicated she is stabilized with no advancing lesions and has returned to work.*

7. —— A *fifty-three-year-old female who came to the clinic in October 1980 with 8 out of 10 positive nodes after a mastectomy in 1979. Postoperatively, she had received radiation for twenty-three days and chemotherapy courses for one year. When her nodes returned she came to the clinic and was put on the standard program of immunotherapy. Her nodes diminished. However, she dropped her program and five months later returned to the clinic with an abdominal mass. Diagnosis revealed a 3-cm mass of bilateral metastatic cancer of both ovaries. We started her on the standard program again and referred her for surgical removal of her ovaries. Echograms indicated she was clear of cancer following our treatment and surgery. A telephone check at the time of this writing indicated she has had no recurrence and is feeling well.*

8. —— A *sixty-four-year-old female who came to the clinic in August 1974 with Level III malignant melanoma of the left*

ankle and groin resection. She responded well to immunotherapy. Tests in 1982 indicated she remains cleared of cancer. She returns for regular checkups and at the time of this writing is still clear.

9. —— *A sixty-five-year-old male who came to the clinic in May 1981 with cancer of the prostate with multiple metastases to the bone (revealed by scan in 1980). On the standard program his prostate mass had gone down by July 1981, and his bone lesions greatly diminished by August 1982. A check with his physician at the time of this writing indicated he is doing well, continuing his vaccines and diet program.*

10. —— *A thirty-three-year-old female who came to the clinic in January 1979 with a diagnosis of Hodgkin's disease. She had had earlier surgical removal of a mass of her right lung, but now periaortic nodules were present. She responded well to the standard program of immunotherapy and remained clear for four years. At the time of this writing we found she'd undergone considerable emotional trauma during the previous six weeks and had had a recurrence in the chest. She will now undergo a course of modified chemotherapy while maintaining her immunity.*

11. —— *A fifty-one-year-old male who came to the clinic in February 1977 with Clark's Level II malignant melanoma of the nodular type in his back, as well as aortic nodes. He had had multiple surgeries to remove nodes. Even after continued recurrences, he responded well to immunotherapy. Radiology reports in February 1983 confirmed that there was no evidence of cancer in his body.*

12. —— *A sixty-eight-year-old female who came to the clinic in September 1980 with tumors of the uterus, a 7-cm tumor of the vagina, and lesions of the liver. After immunization, we referred her to a local hospital in San Diego for small doses of chemotherapy and radiation. Ultrasound and scans in February 1981 indicated the tumor and lesions were diminishing. She re-*

turned to New York to resume her career. A recent check with her New York physician indicates that while not completely clear she is doing well. Previous to therapy she weighed 80 pounds (36 kg) and was a total invalid. Presently she weighs 120 pounds (54 kg) and is working.

13. —— A sixty-seven-year-old female who came to the clinic in June 1976 with a pathology report of two positive masses in her breasts. She had refused a mastectomy, but after diagnosis at the clinic we recommended surgical removal of the masses, followed by the standard program of immunotherapy. When she returned to the clinic in February 1983 for tests, she was still clear.

14. —— A sixty-three-year-old female who came to the clinic in June 1972 for preventive care following radiation and a right radical mastectomy with two positive nodes. In 1975 she developed hypercalcemia (an excess of calcium in the blood). A parathyroid adenoma was found and surgically removed. She has had no recurrence and at the time of this writing she remains well.

15. —— A thirty-eight-year-old female who came to the clinic in February 1974 with widespread cancer of the abdomen following surgery in January of 1973 for adenocarcinoma and bilateral involvement of the ovaries with attachment to the uterus. Radiation followed surgery, but the cancer had spread to her scarred underlying tissue. At the clinic she followed our immunotherapy. In 1978 ultrasound showed no metastases, no fluid, and that her liver was clear; a 1981 chest X ray was normal. A pelvic examination and echograms at the time of this writing indicated she is still clear of cancer.

16. —— A fifty-five-year-old female who came to the clinic in June 1976 with a diagnosis of terminal lymphoma (Hodgkin's disease). Pleural effusion and a 6 cm × 5 cm periaortic node were present, as well as liver metastasis. She underwent immuno-

therapy and stabilized in 1978. Echograms in 1980 indicated that she was free of cancer, and her nodes normal. In 1982 ultrasound indicated her liver was normal with no masses. A recent office visit at the time of this writing revealed she is still clear of cancer but has developed cardiac angina and heart disease.

17. —— *A seventy-six-year-old female who came to the clinic in March of 1976 after a radical mastectomy for poorly differentiated carcinoma of the breast, followed by 4 out of 12 nodes tested positive for cancer. She underwent the standard program of immunotherapy, and by the end of 1976 a complete checkup indicated that she was clear. A telephone report at the time of this writing indicated she is still healthy and doing well. She received no radiation or chemotherapy.*

18. —— *A sixty-six-year-old male who came to the clinic in June 1978 with inoperable cancer of the right kidney with metastasis to the liver and a massive retro-peritoneal lesion from the liver to the pelvis. He had received some radiation but stopped it and came to the clinic. In 1979 he was feeling much better, and in 1980 his tumor had diminished from 8 cm to 4 cm. By 1981 his cancer had stabilized. A telephone check at the time of this writing indicated he was still on his program and doing well.*

19. —— *A forty-one-year-old male who came to the clinic in August 1973 with a diagnosis of Level IV melanoma of the right thigh with metastatic nodes in the groin removed by surgery. He responded well to the standard program of immunotherapy. A punch biopsy in January of 1983 at UCLA indicated he is still totally free of cancer.*

20. —— *A fifty-year-old female who came to the clinic in June of 1977 with infiltrative lobular carcinoma of the right breast and two positive axillary nodes. She had refused both surgery and chemotherapy. We put her on the standard program of immu-*

notherapy. Echograms in 1979 showed that she had cleared. However, while traveling for two years she went off the program and relapsed. She returned to the clinic in 1981 with cancer spread to the chest wall and pathological confirmation of positive neck nodes. She began immunotherapy again, and echograms at the time of this writing show that she is now cleared.

21. —— *A twenty-one-year-old male who came to the clinic in January 1976 with Hodgkin's disease, positive nodes in the neck and metastasis to the bone. He had undergone three courses of chemotherapy during a four month period but stopped treatments prior to arriving at the clinic. He had also had his spleen removed. We treated him with the standard program of immunotherapy. An ultrasound in 1981 showed him clear of metastases. The last time he was seen for examination, in September of 1982, all scans were negative.*

22. —— *A seventy-two-year-old female who came to the clinic in August 1974 with malignant melanoma on her back and positive nodes under the left arm. She underwent our standard program of immunotherapy. An ultrasound in 1981 showed her clear, and echograms and scans in May 1982 indicated she was clear with no recurrence. A visit to the clinic just prior to the time of this writing showed her still clear.*

23. —— *A seventy-one-year-old male who came to the clinic in November 1977 following removal of a tumor of the colon and a pathology report showing positive nodes with metastasis to the omentum. He responded well to the standard program of immunotherapy. An ultrasound in 1980 showed no evidence of new lesions and no enlargements of old lesions. A check with his family physician at the time of this writing confirms he is clear today and feeling well.*

24. —— *A sixty-nine-year-old female who came to the clinic in December 1975 with a pathological diagnosis of poorly*

differentiated adenocarcinoma of the breast with metastasis to surrounding nodes following a modified mastectomy the previous year. She refused further surgery and underwent our standard program of immunotherapy. A bone scan was negative in 1981. Regular office checkups up to the time of this writing confirm she is still clear with no recurrence.

25. —— *A fifty-five-year-old female who came to the clinic in September 1979 with squamous cell carcinoma of the larynx confirmed by biopsy. We referred her for mild radiation and gave her simultaneous immunization with the standard program of immunotherapy. A laryngoscopic examination of her throat in April 1982 showed no malignancy.*

26. —— *A sixty-one-year-old female who came to the clinic in April of 1980 with a pathology report of Grade III intraductal cell carcinoma and metastasis to the right lobe of liver. She had had a lumpectomy in March 1980 and refused further surgery, radiation, and chemotherapy. We treated her with the standard program of immunotherapy and as of October 1982 echograms showed she was clear of cancer. Telephone follow-up at the time of this writing confirmed she is still well.*

27. —— *A twenty-five-year-old male who came to the clinic in June 1976 with Hodgkin's disease and 128 subcutaneous skin lesions of his neck and back complicated by severe allergies. He responded well when treated with immunotherapy plus surgical removal of some of the nodes. Unfortunately, he refuses to maintain his program of vaccines and diet but comes back to the clinic whenever he discovers a new lesion, at which point we reinstitute our program. At his last visit at the time of this writing, he has a small lesion supraclavicular left neck, now receding. His health is otherwise good.*

28. —— *A forty-three-year-old male who came to the clinic in January 1981 for preventive therapy after surgery for the*

removal of a cancerous kidney. He responded well to our standard program of immunotherapy. He was seen in July 1982, and there was no further incidence of cancer.

29. —— A *sixty-seven-year-old male who came to the clinic in February 1982 with a huge (18 cm × 22 cm) chondrosarcoma of the right buttock. He had had radiation and chemotherapy, but the mass had continued to grow. At the clinic we referred him for surgical removal and treated him with immunotherapy. A recent check confirms that there has been no recurrence, and that he is completely normal.*

30. —— A *twelve-year-old male who came to the clinic in April 1981 with advanced Hodgkin's disease, and whose mother had refused chemotherapy for him. He had developed a heart murmur and a lesion on his liver. The court was threatening to take the child away from his mother because she had refused the chemotherapy. I informed the court that he was under our care; the mother was then allowed to keep him, and we began treatments. In January 1982 an ultrasound indicated lymphoma (a tumor of the lymphoid tissues) in remission. A recent check confirmed that he is totally clear, back in school, gaining weight, and at the time of this writing has made the basketball team.*

31. —— A *fifty-one-year-old female who came to the clinic in February 1981 with cancer of the ovaries with metastasis of a baseball-size tumor on the colon which had been surgically removed. She also had had a small node on the back of her neck removed. She had had 3,000 rads of radiation and two treatments of chemotherapy with Alkaran. She stopped the chemotherapy treatments because she was so sick. Her physician's report at the time she came to the clinic described her as "terminal." We treated her with immunotherapy, and in 1982 a pelvic and abdominal CAT scan was negative and an ultrasound was normal. At the time of this writing all scans were negative, and she was back at work.*

32. —— A sixty-seven-year-old female who came to the clinic in June 1977 with adenocarcinoma of the endometrium (the mucous membrane lining the uterus) with metastasis to the liver and having had a hysterectomy and radiation. A postoperative biopsy report revealed eight lesions approximately 4 cm × 4 cm in the right lobe of the liver and positive nodes in the inguinal (groin) region. The patient refused further surgery and was treated with our program. As of October 1979 both nodes and liver lesions were proved cleared by scans. Telephone checkup at the time of this writing indicated she is still clear.

33. —— A sixty-seven-year-old male who came to the clinic in May 1979 with cancer of the pancreas and metastasis to the liver. He had originally been admitted to the hospital with severe abdominal pain. Initial studies showed it to be pancreatitis, but an upper GI series then revealed evidence of a mass lesion. A CAT scan showed a fairly extensive tumor of the pancreas involving the liver. The patient was told he had six weeks to live. He refused chemotherapy and came to the clinic. We treated him with immunotherapy and in May 1981 CAT, bone, and liver scans showed the tumor was in remission and the liver lesion decreased. A biopsy in February 1982 showed the liver normal.

34. —— A forty-four-year-old female who came to the clinic in January 1981 with Paget's disease of the breast and bleeding from the nipple. She had refused removal of the breast and underwent our program of immunotherapy. The surface of the nipple cleared but a biopsy revealed some malignant cells. She was undecided whether to have a mastectomy, as urged by her oncologist in 1983. A telephone check at the time of this writing revealed she had the mastectomy, which showed her breast and axilla completely clear with only a few superficial neoplastic cells.

35. —— A forty-three-year-old female who came to the clinic in January 1977 after discovering a nodule in her right

breast. It was diagnosed as malignant and a mastectomy rec-
ommended. The patient preferred a lumpectomy, which she had.
Afterward, we treated her with our program of immunotherapy,
but she discontinued it. In January of 1978 she had a recurrence
and a mastectomy. A pathology report revealed an infiltrating
ductal-type carcinoma with 5 out of 12 positive nodes in the axilla
(armpit), estrogen positive, and an ovarian tumor. She had a
modified hysterectomy and an oophorectomy (removal of the ova-
ries) in 1979 after resuming immunotherapy at the clinic. In
February 1982 a mammogram showed no further metastases and
no new nodes.

     36. —— *A fifty-two-year-old female who came to the clinic*
in March 1980 following a hysterectomy for adenocarcinoma of
the uterus with postoperative diagnosis of bilateral metastases to
the pelvis and omentum. She could not take BCG vaccinations
because of a positive skin test, but we treated her with autogenous
vaccines and antibiotics, intravenous vitamin C, and diet ther-
apy. She cleared by April 1981. In May of 1982 ultrasound showed
there was no evidence of mass or lesions.

     37. —— *A seventy-three-year-old male who came to the*
clinic in October 1977 following removal of the upper lobe of the
right lung for cancer, with a subsequent pathology report showing
metastasis to the peribronchial lymph nodes and to the liver. He
received our program of immunotherapy and in March of 1979
X rays, ultrasound, scans, and blood chemistry showed he was
completely free of cancer. He continues to be clear at the time of
this writing.

     38. —— *A forty-eight-year-old female who came to the*
clinic in September 1978 with part of her liver and one third of
her colon removed. She was reported to have residual metastases.
We treated her with our program of immunotherapy, and in 1979
she stabilized. In December 1981 an ultrasound showed a normal

liver and no evidence of cancer in the colon. A telephone conversation at the time of this writing indicated she is still clear.

39. —— *A thirty-seven-year-old female who came to the clinic in June 1981 with recurring tumors in the pelvic region. She had had pelvic masses which were biopsied as lymphomas in 1976 with surgical removal followed by three and a half years of chemotherapy. When tumors continued to grow, she stopped the chemotherapy and we treated her with our program of immunotherapy. One year later, ultrasound showed the tumors had decreased. At the time of this writing ultrasound showed a total absence of any masses and that she is free of cancer.*

40. —— *A sixty-four-year-old female who came to the clinic in August 1981 with advanced cancer of the breast and twenty-eight positive nodes and metastasis to bone and liver. An intensive immunotherapy program stabilized her, but the clinic suddenly lost contact with her. A telephone check with a close relative at the time of this writing indicated she had stopped her vaccines and diet in May of 1982 and died peacefully in her sleep of heart failure at the end of that year.*

41. —— *A sixty-year-old male who came to the clinic in July 1975 having had a resection for cancer of the colon. He had metastasis to the liver and spine. This patient was a medical doctor who refused chemotherapy and radiation when he appeared at our clinic. We treated him with immunotherapy. A telephone check at the time of this writing confirmed that he is still completely recovered and active in his retirement.*

42. —— *A sixty-year-old female who came to the clinic in August 1979, referred to us as "terminal" by her doctor, who had given her two to three weeks to live. She suffered from cancer of the esophagus and liver metastasis. She had had part of her stomach removed and nine months of chemotherapy. We treated her with immunotherapy, and at the time of this writing, three*

and a half years later, she is still alive, has gained five pounds, and is doing well. A recent CAT scan was negative, and signs of cancer are clear.

43. —— *A sixty-seven-year-old male who came to the clinic in October 1981 with metastatic cancer of the prostate, bones, bladder, and a large chest mass with rib destruction and right lung involvement. We treated him with immunotherapy, and at the time of this writing all scans are negative. His own physician also reports all cancer signs clear and scans negative.*

44. —— *A seventy-year-old female who came to the clinic in November 1981, having had a mastectomy for infiltrating carcinoma of the left breast. We treated her preventively with the standard program of immunotherapy, and at the time of this writing she is still on the program and free of cancer.*

45. —— *A seventy-one-year-old female who came to the clinic in July 1977 with a twenty-year history of recurring basal cell carcinoma on her face that had been periodically removed with cauterizations and surgeries. We put her on a prevention program. Except for two growths removed in October and December of 1981, she has had no recurrences. She continues with a modified immunotherapy program.*

46. —— *A sixty-three-year-old female who came to the clinic in August 1981, diagnosed as "terminal" by her physician after having had colon surgery the previous March with a postoperative pathology report of widespread metastasis to the bones and an additional 4-cm mass recurring on the colon. We treated her with immunotherapy, and at the time of this writing her scans are still positive. She has had a recent colostomy and will have to have radiation. We are hopeful she will continue to survive.*

47. —— *A forty-three-year-old female who came to the clinic in August 1979 with recurring nodules after having had*

modified mastectomies of the right breast in January and the left breast in July. She had come for preventive treatment and underwent our program. Tests at the end of August 1982 showed that her nodules had diminished and there was no further recurrence. We have not heard from her since.

48. ———— A fifty-year-old female who came to the clinic in February 1982 with breast cancer and metastatic lung disease. She had undergone a radical mastectomy, after which dozens of nodes appeared under her arms, across her chest and over her spine. During radiation her pericardium (the membranous sac enclosing the heart) was burned so severely that she developed pericarditis, necessitating puncturing and draining the pericardium. Chemotherapy had no effect on the growth of her nodules initially. When this patient appeared at the clinic she carried oxygen and could not walk more than two or three steps without having to stop and use it. We immediately put her on a strong immunization program. We also referred her for modified chemotherapy and additional but minimal radiation. At the time of this writing scans and echograms indicate she is totally clear. On the morning of her last visit she had jogged two miles on the San Diego beach. Her future, however, is uncertain because of continued chemotherapy.

49. ———— A fifty-seven-year-old female who came to the clinic in October 1978 with cancer of the breast and bone cancer of the left hip. She had had a hysterectomy and an oophorectomy (removal of the ovaries) in 1966 and 1967, respectively, before coming to the clinic. We treated her with immunotherapy. A scan in 1979 and another at the end of 1982 showed no evidence of cancer.

50. ———— A sixty-two-year-old female who came to the clinic in July 1981 after having had a hysterectomy and mastectomy for adenocarcinoma of the right breast, Stage II, followed by che-

motherapy. The chemotherapy was too toxic; during this time there was widespread recurrence of nodes with 17 of 26 nodes positive and a large two-inch tumor in her axilla. We treated her with immunotherapy. At the time of this writing scans and a physical examination indicate she is clear.

51. —— A forty-five-year-old female who came to the clinic in October 1981 with malignant Level III melanoma of the right buttock. After surgical removal and treatment with immuno-therapy she has become completely clear as confirmed by a tele-phone call to her physician at the time of this writing. She remains on the prevention program.

52. —— A sixty-three-year-old female who came to the clinic in December 1981 after a left radical mastectomy, including removal of six positive nodes. We put her on prevention therapy, and she has recently developed small nodes under her scar. She is still on the program. An X ray in November 1982 revealed no metastasis. In February 1983 her lumps were diminishing.

53. —— A fifty-five-year-old female who came to the clinic in November 1981. She was diagnosed as having a 2.5 cm × 2.8 cm tumor of the left lung, lower lobe, which was metastatic to 5 of 7 nodes in the area. The September before she came to the clinic, the lobe was removed. A body scan showed bones, liver, and spleen in good condition. The patient had never smoked but had been around heavy smokers all her life. She had neither ra-diation nor chemotherapy. In February 1982 a chest X ray showed no pleural effusion. She is currently following the program, and a recent chest X ray at the time of this writing showed no evidence of recurrence.

54. —— A sixty-two-year-old female who came to the clinic in October 1981 having been declared "terminal" by her physician with cancer of the colon and an extremely large metastasis to her

liver. She also had heart problems. She stayed alive for a full year on our program of immunotherapy, but we suddenly lost contact with her at the end of 1982. She is presumed dead.

55. —— *A sixty-six-year-old female who came to the clinic in June 1981 with cancer of the breasts with metastasis to the ribs. Radiation had no effect but to break down the skin on the wall of her chest. We put her on full immunotherapy. At the end of 1982 echograms, X rays, and scans showed marked improvement. Only one bad spot in the rib remains.*

56. —— *A sixty-four-year-old male physician who came to the clinic in January 1980 with cancer of the prostate and basal cell cancer of the face. This patient refused radiation or chemotherapy and was concerned because several members of his family had died of cancer. We put him on the regular program, and tests in January of 1982 indicated he was clear of cancer. A telephone check at the time of this writing confirmed he is still clear.*

57. —— *A fifty-five-year-old female who came to the clinic in September 1976 after a hysterectomy and with metastasis to the pelvis. She had refused surgery. Chemotherapy resulted in no improvement. After radiation made her severely sick she terminated both treatments and came to us with a recurrent inoperable mass in her rectum. At the clinic we discovered an inoperable 12 cm × 12 cm tumor between her vagina and rectum. At the time of this writing, after almost seven years, she is not completely well and remains under treatment. The mass has been reduced to one-fourth its former size, and she seems to be progressing slowly and is living a normal life.*

58. —— *A seventy-year-old male who came to the clinic in January 1981 with oat-cell cancer of the lung and right neck metastasis. He responded well to immunotherapy. He contacted us in February 1982 and said he was doing well and that his*

doctors couldn't believe his improvement. This man subsequently died, but there is little doubt that our program prolonged his life at least an additional year.

59. —— *A twenty-six-year-old female who came to the clinic in June 1981 with a malignant melanoma of the forehead that spread to the right lung and bones. She had had extensive chemotherapy and radiation and went on and off our immunotherapy program at the clinic, never remaining with any one therapy for any length of time. She died in 1982.*

60. —— *A sixty-six-year-old female who came to the clinic in August 1978 with a lymphoma of the small bowel with metastases to the spleen and aorta. She was declared inoperable and "terminal" by her physician after she failed to respond to radiation. We began strong immunotherapy. After the patient started to respond she moved from New York City to San Diego to be close to the clinic. Scans, ultrasound, and blood chemistries at the time of this writing indicate that she is completely clear of cancer and leading a normal life.*

61. —— *A sixty-year-old female who came to the clinic in April 1982. In 1980 she had had a radical mastectomy with nearly all nodes (31 of 32) positive and was treated with chemotherapy. She had also had cancer of the ribs and sternum treated with 3000 rads of radiation in September and July 1981. The front of her right breast was inflamed. As we treated her, she improved. In October 1982 her bone scan was negative, and she went home. Unfortunately, she reactivated and came back in poor condition. She started on the program again, and improved. However, she went on and off our program, and died.*

62. —— *A forty-seven-year-old female who came to the clinic in November 1979 with cancer of the breast with metastases to the scapula and adrenals, a mass in her uterus, and infiltration*

in both lungs. She had had a mastectomy in 1972, an oophorectomy (removal of the ovaries), and then an adrenalectomy in 1979, and several courses of chemotherapy. When she appeared at the clinic she had developed lesions of her pelvis. We treated her with the usual immunotherapy. In 1982 ultrasound showed her lesions diminishing and her chest clear. A telephone check at the time of this writing indicates she is completely clear and feeling fine.

With the approval of the patient, we will provide access to photocopies of any patient's chart to any licensed physician or qualified researcher. Also with patient approval, we will put such qualified investigators in touch with the patient for personal interview. The clinic is open for inspection or educational visit to any physician, prospective patient, or representative of an accredited institution.

As always, we invite any member of the American Cancer Society or the National Cancer Institute to make a careful investigation of our clinic, our program, and our results with cancer patients.

3

THE ORTHODOX CANCER THERAPIES

ARE THE TREATMENTS WORSE THAN THE DISEASE?

Much of what is done in the treatment of cancer by surgery, irradiation and chemotherapy represents halfway technology in the sense that these measures are directed at the existence of already established cancer cells, but not at the mechanisms by which cells become neoplastic.

LEWIS THOMAS
Lives of a Cell: Notes of a Biology Watcher

THE OLD JOKE about good news and bad news applies to the person who has just found out he has cancer. The good news, as our random case histories show, is that in most cases you can strengthen your immune system and recover from this horrible disease. That is, just as with smallpox, TB, and polio, there is an immunotherapy protocol that can save your life.

The bad news is that you will probably be talked into undergoing one of the three orthodox treatments of cancer before you finally realize that these treatments frequently can be more deadly than the disease itself.

This is because each one of them, to one degree or another, is aimed at the destruction of the cancer cell (as well as surrounding healthy cells) and not at the *cause* of it. Each treatment attacks the manifestation of the disease, without working to prevent it. It's a lot like shooting mad dogs, but ignoring a cure for rabies.

These orthodox treatments are:

■ *surgery* (cut out the tumor and hope it won't grow back or pop up somewhere else);

■ *radiation* (destroy the tumor with sharply focused high doses of radiation, and hope you don't simultaneously destroy the patient's vital tissues surrounding it);

■ *chemotherapy* (introduce certain highly toxic chemicals into the patient's system and hope they'll attack the tumor and kill it before they kill the patient.)

All of these treatments are drastic measures necessitated by drastic situations, and even though they each offer a certain degree of hope to the desperate patient, they also set up terrible anxieties. These anxieties are justified. While there are statistics that show how each of these treatments has achieved some measure of remission (notice I didn't say "cure"), each also suppresses the immune system's ability to function properly in the life or death battle against the disease. Each treatment can also reduce the patient's ability or desire to eat and thereby undermine the body's nutritional requirements in arming the immune system for a long, drawn-out struggle.

So here we are with a vicious circle that can be, and most frequently is, fatal to the patient. The other old saw also becomes true: The operation was a success, but the patient died. The treatment is worse than the disease, and the patient literally dies from it and not from the cancer. The treatment harms the immune system, which needs nutrients to fight back. Yet due to the treatment the patient is often unable or doesn't want to eat. The lack of nutrients further undermines the immune system, requiring additional treatment, and so on until the cancer eventually wins the fight. Further, even while the immune system is starved for nutrients, the chemicals from chemotherapy, the tissue destruction from radiation, and the trauma of surgery are all keeping the immune system from fighting the cancer cells off, just as surely as if some traitorous munitions maker had outfitted the "good guys" with blank ammunition before they went into battle. The black hats win, because the white hats were helpless without reinforcements.

Dr. Richard O. Brennan, medical director of the Bellevue Metabolic Clinic of Houston and founder of the International Academy of Preventive Medicine, puts it very succinctly in his book, *Coronary? Cancer? God's Answer: Prevent It!* (Harvest House, 1979):

Our cancer research is misdirected, inefficient, and inadequate. We have almost as many people living off the disease as are dying from it. The government spends billions on cancer research, but at the same time allows known carcinogens in our processed foods, subsidizes cigarettes, and continues to develop new radiation, surgical, and chemotherapy techniques when burning, cutting, and poisoning have already proved largely unsuccessful. Physicians have not been trained in preventive medicine and, not having experience or knowledge of preventive medicine, they continue the outmoded but orthodox approach of treating symptoms rather than the entire body.

Let's examine each of the orthodox treatments separately and evaluate its effectiveness. It is my contention that, if you asked an honest oncologist for the truth, you would be told that only 15 to 20 percent of all patients derive any benefit from his treatments. Hence, it is important for you to know exactly what you can rightfully expect when you are faced with these orthodox treatments as explained by an establishment physician.

Surgery. Let me first say that surgery has a definite place in the immunotherapy approach to cancer treatment. It is recommended frequently at our clinic, because, when possible, it is best to remove large masses of cancerous cells from the patient (called "debulking") in order to give the immune system a head start in its comeback fight against the disease. When you have a tumor of billions of cancerous cells multiplying frightfully fast, you are asking a lot of the immune system to "catch up" after the cancer has been decimating your own cells for months or even years. In short, surgery can reduce the number of men in black hats.

The thing most surgeons and cancer physicians do not understand yet is that cancer is a *systemic* disease. The tumor is only a symptom of the disease; the disease causes the tumor, not vice versa. Frequently, after a surgeon has cut out a tumor and made a wide dissection, one hears that he "got it all." This is supposed to be good news—and indeed the surgeon announces it enthusiastically enough—but in the majority of cases nothing is subsequently done to raise the patient's immunity. There will probably be a recurrence of cancer within a few months or years.

In other words, this first line of defense can sometimes be effective in *postponing* the deadly growth of more cancer, but most often the patient is so stressed by the trauma of the procedure that he or she never fully recovers. Chances for recovery are worsened by the fact that even after surgery the patient still has the disease. The immune system needs to be strengthened to its maximum in order to fight off the cancer.

If a lesion is a local one, accessible to surgery, then removal might be helpful. Sometimes, when the entire tumor cannot be resected, removal of even part of it may give the body a chance to cooperate in eliminating the rest of the residual tumor.

Yet in may cases, including some in which the patient refused surgery, we have achieved great success in beginning immunotherapy treatments immediately and continuing until finally the patient's own immune system has attacked the tumor and completely eliminated it. This, of course, is in early detection of cancer and before a patient has been radiated or given chemotherapy.

Radiation. This method of treatment was thought by many people in the early days to be a great boon to medicine. As better equipment was developed, specialists theorized that radiating the entire body was beneficial to destroying the seeds of cancer. Even today, radiation is held in high regard. Indeed, sometimes radiation at a single point, with a single, sharply focused beam, may help the patient *in one particular spot*. (This is called "spot radiation.") But there is danger as well. Since the bombing of Hiroshima and Nagasaki in August 1945, the more astute cancer researchers have become convinced of one inalterable fact: Radiation destroys human tissues. Not only that, but radiation destroys human tissues forever. Consider what's going on in the front pages of the nation's newspapers today. Nuclear plants malfunction, and the incidence of cancer increases in the community. Radiation exposure during the postwar nuclear tests at Eniwetok Island is proved to be the cause of bone and other cancers in veterans. Diagnostic X rays, considered the innocuous standby of doctors the world over, have come under severe cancer-causing scrutiny.

Does it make sense then to radiate a person who already has cancer? Should it not be used with only the greatest discrimination?

The body is a compact system. It is extremely difficult to radiate that one specific spot with one focused beam without involving neighboring cells—maybe vital cells. If you radiate the rectum or colon, you radiate a lot of the lower bowel. If you radiate the lung, you're going to get the ribs and the esophagus and the trachea and the bronchii. It's not a simple procedure, and its success rate is not high. Radiation still has only minimal beneficial effects in the treatment of cancer.

Radiation has a remarkable ability to surpress immunity. It's been shown in many laboratory and clinical studies that, following a large dose of X rays over the entire body, animals and human beings become susceptible to infections and may die from them in spite of intensive antibiotic therapy. Also, the ability of the body to manufacture immune-producing cells may be permanently inhibited. Nowhere is the immune-suppressant effect of radiation so dramatically demonstrated as in the fact that radiation in combination with certain chemicals is being used prior to organ transplant surgery. The patient's immune system is so lowered in strength by the radiation that the body doesn't reject the organ as readily, and the chances of success are greater. This, of course, may be one of the benefits of radiation, but the patient's immune system must thereafter be rescued.

Chemotherapy. A very wise physician in San Francisco, Dr. Collin H. Dong, who has been very successful in treating arthritis with biological methods, once said: "Chemicals and drugs only make a battlefield out of your body. And when was the last time you saw anything beautiful growing on a battlefield?"

This is the chief problem with chemotherapy. The drugs and chemicals introduced into your system are so toxic, so deadly to cells and tissues, that while they may be doing some good against the cells of a tumor, they are most assuredly weakening your immune system simultaneously. And what is the sense in destroying a tumor, achieving a temporary remission, if you are left with an immune system so damaged that another tumor—or the same one—can grow back? At first glance it may appear to the physician that these cell poisons, although they don't necessarily prolong life, may relieve some of the *symptoms* of cancer in some patients. But it is only at the cost of the destruction of the regenerative powers of the patient's immune system.

Often patients who are immune competent, i.e., capable of making immune, defensive agents, become incapable of doing so under chemical treatment. If chemotherapy is recommended, it's worth it to find out if the patient is immune competent. Extensive studies of the ability of patients to be immunized against various agents should be undertaken, as well as studies of their cellular response to treatment. And since this response is so variable, it is impossible for the average physician who administers chemotherapeutic drugs to know exactly what is happening. He is guided by a rule of thumb—the number of white cells circulating in the blood as shown by the blood count, and the condition of the bone marrow as shown by a bone marrow biopsy. Generally, the immunocompetence of the patient remains an unknown factor. One of the great problems facing the average physician today is how to evaluate a patient's response to chemical therapy and protect against injury to the immune system. Only at large medical centers under expert supervision can the variations in immunocompetence be evaluated. Usually, patients are referred to a specialist, probably an oncologist. The problem is that many oncologists know little more than the average physician about the science of immunology, which is practically nothing.

What can be said in a positive way about these orthodox treatments? Only these two things in general:

1. Each can be temporarily useful in *most* cases, and somewhat more effective in *some* cases. Surgery can remove *some* tumors. Radiation and chemotherapy can diminish *some* tumors.
2. The effectiveness of each orthodox therapy can be increased, sometimes multiplied, when accompanied by a sound nutritional support program designed to boost the immune system. (A San Diego oncologist with whom we work closely reports that patients whom we have already put on a sound nutritional and immunological regimen have an exceptionally higher rate of recovery than his other patients.)

Conventional treatments, as they exist today, are fundamentally self-defeating. Obviously, the key to the effective treatment of cancer lies in enhancing the immune system, not in suppressing it. If a patient's immune system is not well fortified and then rigorously maintained, the chances of survival are slim.

It is well known that the effect of certain chemotherapeutic drugs on the immune system is so severe that *new* areas of cancer may appear during or soon after the treatment designed to eradicate the old cancer. Finally, irradiation and chemotherapy patients often have their immune systems so destroyed that they contract infectious diseases, such as pneumonia, from which they die before the cancer has a chance to kill them.

There is no doubt that the effectiveness of these treatments depends a great deal upon what immunological precautions are taken simultaneously. A nutritional program restores immune function, aids in forestalling further outbreaks of cancer and other infections, and prevents excessive weight loss. Moreover, our studies have repeatedly shown that patients who switch completely from orthodox treatment, chemotherapy for example, to nutritional immunotherapy significantly increase their chances of eliminating cancer from their bodies completely. Or, at the very least, their life expectancy increases to a greater degree than those patients treated only with chemotherapy.

Nutrition-based immunotherapy is free of the troublesome side effects that occur in all three orthodox treatments. It is not a debilitating method of treating cancer, and it is in no way harmful to the body.

Ultimately, the best method of treating cancer is to prevent it. And this, at last, is possible for everyone.

We have reached a point in medical history where we are so technologically sophisticated, so well endowed with the greatest of investigative research instruments, that we are almost morally obliged to investigate alternatives to the orthodox techniques that are proving so ineffective. There is a great deal of important new work being done that can save millions of lives, and yet much of it is being politically suppressed.

We have all heard the litany of far-thinking, intuitive scientists whose research observations and clinical findings leap-frogged ahead of contemporary orthodox thinking, but who were cast out from society and the scientific community for daring to present their theories. Copernicus and Galileo were threatened with imprisonment and torture unless they recanted their theories. A simple country doctor named Edward Jenner observed that milkmaids who contracted cowpox were somehow immunized against smallpox. When he vaccinated some of his young patients with a cowpox vaccine, and they didn't contract smallpox, Jenner, who is now considered the father of immunology, was attacked by medical authorities because he couldn't explain *why* his vaccine worked. Pasteur, who further refined Jenner's work with his anthrax and rabies vaccines, and who actually brought the new science of immunization to the world at large by his insistence upon the existence of organisms "too small to be seen," was ridiculed for most of his life—after all, he was a chemist, not a doctor! From Paracelsus (1493–1531) to Semmelweis (1818–1865), doctors railed against the "establishments" of their day for clinging to ideas that were actually killing patients. It more than 400 years to convince surgeons to wash their hands before entering the operating room.

There are similar pioneers alive today, working at the cutting edge of medical innovation and scientific discovery. Certain vaccines against cancer have been available for more than 100 years yet are suppressed at every turn by American special interests within the establishment hierarchy. Brilliant researchers abroad have been refused entry into this country; others have been forced to move to Canada or the Bahamas. And when the words "nutrition," "bacteria," or "vaccine" are mentioned in connection with the prevention and treatment of cancer, many physicians and surgeons wince and turn their well-trained heads from such "quackery," refusing even to examine the evidence. There is an old saying that might apply: "Doctors are always down on something they're not up on."

Perhaps the story of my own husband, Dr. Owen Webster Wheeler, will demonstrate more dramatically than any other what I mean by investigating new ideas before deciding on an established treatment for cancer. He is a medical doctor who practiced for more than thirty years in the city of San Diego and was one of the founders of Doctors Hospital in that city. (We were both married to different spouses at the time his story begins and were not acquainted with each other.)

DR. OWEN W. WHEELER'S STORY

I was shaving one morning when my wife happened to notice a lump on the side and to the rear of my neck, just above the clavicle. I hadn't noticed it before but upon examining it, my training told me something was terribly wrong. I knew what it was, but I didn't want to admit it to myself. "Hm, some kind of lump," I said to my wife, and finished dressing.

That afternoon I went to a surgeon friend, to whom I had referred hundreds of patients from my family practice, and with whom I had assisted at hundreds of operations. He took a biopsy. The report he handed me days later said exactly what I feared it would—cancer. There was no question. Furthermore, he told me it was inoperable, as it was close to the carotid artery and probably attached to it, as well as being wrapped around important nerves and blood vessels.

I sat down and said nothing for a long while. Physicians, when they start their medical practice and throughout their professional careers, take vaccinations and inoculations because they are exposed to disease all the time; usually, they stay well. I never thought I would get cancer, although I'd been around it so often. "What should I do? What should I do?" was all I could say. I was afraid.

My friend the surgeon advised me that the standard radiation and chemotherapy techniques were my only hope since no one would operate. Without them, he said, I had no chance to survive for more than a year.

I remember sitting down one evening and wondering whether I would be alive in a year, whether, if I were, I'd be a skeleton in some hospital bed. My wife and I cried. And we prayed.

A physician sees cancer all the time. We read about it, we see other doctors' patients, we discover it in our own patients, and we hear about it in the medical meetings we are always attending. And we always advise the orthodox treatments. We have to, of course. A physician could lose his license if he ordered a cancer treatment other than surgery, radiation, or chemotherapy.

I finally called an old friend, a local oncologist to whom I'd referred many patients. He agreed with the surgeon, that the tumor—it was the size of a lemon—was completely inoperable because it was surrounding so many nerves and blood vessels and was touching the top of one lung. I knew if this person couldn't "get it all," as they say, no one could. He was one of the best.

I did a strange thing at this time. At least, it seems strange now. I had been referring cancer patients not only to this oncologist but to several others for many years, and it suddenly occurred to me that I hadn't ever seen many of those patients again. I called the various specialists, and discovered that most of my patients had died. I thought of my father who had died of cancer a number of years earlier. Nothing the doctors had done had been able to save his life. And the tragedy was that at the autopsy it was determined that there was no cancer left in him. He was rid of the cancer and had been killed by generalized infection due to immune suppression.

I decided that I didn't want to be treated with radiation or chemotherapy. It struck me as curious that for years I'd been referring patients for radiation and chemotherapy procedures, and now I was reluctant to undergo them myself. I had been recommending treatments that seldom cured! Why do oncologists keep administering the same treatments over and over again when they rarely work? I began to feel guilty. Why did I, a physician/healer, recommend that my patients subject themselves to useless "cures"?

I decided to investigate what was being done in alternative cancer therapy. I was looking for people who were doing something other than what I'd been advising for the past ten or fifteen years. I was only sixty-two at the time and wanted to live a few more years.

A friend finally said, "Why don't you look in your own back-yard? There's the Livingston Clinic here in San Diego and they're doing something with cancer patients." I hadn't heard anything about the clinic. I called and made an appointment, and when I got there "Dr. Virginia" took my history. She commented on the fact that I was a physician who was willing to look at alternative therapies and pointed out that, at the time, there had only been a few other physicians to visit the clinic before me.

Dr. Virginia showed me around the laboratory, explained to me her work with the dark-field microscope, and gave me some of her published papers to read. I read about her pioneering work in microbiology and bacteriology, as well as her discoveries of the cancer-causing Progenitor Cryptocides microbe and the hormone that it secreted. I finally saw the microbe in my own blood sample under the dark-field microscope. It was more exciting to me than anything an astronaut circling the moon could have imagined. I felt I was becoming a part of medical history.

As a physician, I had to admit that this approach was completely new to me. Nothing in the literature and the standard cancer information that was being published indicated that anyone was immunizing against cancer. Dr. Virginia explained in detail how the first vaccine, the BCG, which was developed for TB, was also effective against cancer when used with her other modalities; how it was possible, by treating my own total immune system, that cancer was a do-it-yourself treatment disease that my own body could fight, but only if my immune system could be strengthened. She also explained that she made an autogenous vaccine from the actual microbe cultured from my own body fluids. I suddenly realized that I was placing my life in the hands of a woman who claimed to have discovered that cancer was caused by a bacterium, not a virus as I had been taught in medical school. A lot of what she was telling me went totally against my professional training. I, and almost every other doctor in the land, had always stated that it was impossible to have such a bug in one's blood and still live.

After looking at the whole treatment process with an open mind, I decided that it made good scientific sense, and I underwent the program. Within five months my tumor was completely gone. There has never been any recurrence, and it has now been more than ten years. I haven't been sick a day since.

Shortly afterward, in 1975, Dr. Virginia's husband, Dr. A. M. Livingston, died. My wife had died six months pre-

viously of heart disease. When Virginia's husband died, she called to ask if I could come and help her run the clinic. The burden of running it single-handedly was too much, and she would have had to close it had she been unable to find another physician suitable to help out. I was then the only doctor who understood what she was doing and who had seen her results firsthand.

I told Dr. Virginia not to close the clinic, that I would help. Any program that could cure me the way it did was bound to help other patients. I started working at the clinic part-time and devoting less and less time to running my own practice. I became so busy at the clinic that I finally resigned from my partnership to work full-time at the clinic. Dr. Virginia and I kept the clinic open, working side by side, continually seeing cancer patients getting well. I also saw Virginia's unexcelled compassion and concern for her patients. A year later we were married.

4

THE DISCOVERY OF THE CANCER MICROBE, I

THE EARLY WORK

DURING A MEETING of the New York Academy of Sciences at the Waldorf-Astoria Hotel in November of 1969, our research team was describing our discovery of the microorganism that causes cancer and was requested to classify it in the proper bacteriological fashion. All microorganisms are classified into groups according to their unique properties. This is called determinative bacteriology. The classification under a specific name is called nomenclature. All microorganisms, as most of us learned in high school science, are classified under an order, a family, a genus, a species, and variants.

Thus the microbial agent we believe to be the causative agent in cancer is properly classified as follows:

ORDER: Actinomycetales
FAMILY: Progenitoraceae
GENUS: *Cryptocides*
SPECIES: *Cryptocides tumefaciens;*
              Cryptocides sclerodermatis (sclerobacillus);
              Cryptocides wilsonii;
VARIANTS: *Hominis, rodentii, avii,* etc.

What all those impressive words add up to is an increasingly definitive description of the specific microbe. *Actinomycetales* means that the microorganism looks like the sun, having rays or armlike processes in its growth after being planted on culture media in a laboratory dish, such as the petri dishes many of us used in high school and college biology. The culture media is simply biological material that acts as the soil in which the organism grows. (Making the organism grow in such a fashion is called a "culture," or "culturing" the organism.)

We called the microorganism *Progenitoraceae*—or *Progenitor*—because it appears to be very primitive in its growth. Forms resembling these organisms have been found in Precambrian rock. Also it is at the source of life, being present in sperm and in developing embryos. Its genus is *Cryptocides*, a combined Greek and Latin word that means "hidden killer." Under "Species" are named the groups which cause specific diseases, such as cancer, scleroderma (a hardening of the skin), and other connective-tissue diseases. And the variants simply mean that it can occur in several different species, such as man, rodents, birds, etc. It is important here to remember that the Actinomycetales group also contains the microorganisms that cause tuberculosis and leprosy.

The discovery of the microbe *Progenitor Cryptocides* as the causative agent in cancer, and the chronology of the development of our theories on how to treat the disease effectively, is an exciting, frustrating, and heartbreaking story. I was fortunate enough to be "in the right place at the right time" quite often. I also had the good fortune to meet some brilliant researchers and cooperative, pioneering scientists who were not afraid to pursue intuitive pathways that went against the mainstream of popular medical theory. Many of these people risked their personal reputations and professional standing by continuing to work toward advancing scientific knowledge. There are thousands of so-called terminal cancer patients who are cancer-free today, living healthy, vital lives, because these people searched for medical truth along the avenues they did, instead of pursuing the safe, well-trod, "orthodox" boulevards of science.

But first, some terms you should know before the story begins. The *P. Cryptocides* is the ancestral, or primordial, hidden killer that we believe to be implicated in the cause of cancer. Initially, we believed it to be a pathogen only, but with time and further study we realized it was an essential but dormant part of all cells, only activated to repair cell damage. After the repair, it returns to a resting state in the healthy cell, where it remains dormant again. A strong immune system controls this process. However, when immunity is suppressed or weakened, it proliferates and allows cancer to gain a foothold, secreting the same choriogonadotropin hormone found in abundance in all tumors. Hence, as explained more fully later, the P.C. microbe is both a "good guy" and a "bad guy," and for this reason is called an Obligate Symbiont.

One of its properties is that of being *acid-fast*, which, also as touched upon elswhere, means that the microorganism is capable of retaining a certain red dye, carbolfushin, after being washed on a microscope slide with an acid alcohol solution (called decolorization). This trait has allowed researchers to differentiate between this organism and others that are harmless. If an organism is acid-fast, it belongs in the Actinomycetales group and is a first cousin of the lepra and tubercle bacilli.

This method of grouping was discovered accidentally by Robert Koch in 1882 when he was studying TB; it enabled him to identify the tubercle bacillus as its cause. When the acid-fast, red-stained organisms are seen in the sputum of a patient, it means that the patient probably has TB. The same method is applied to nasal smears and tissue preparations from those suspected of having leprosy.

Koch's subsequent work in inoculating TB patients was at first met with scorn by the established medical community, causing heated medical debate. However, in 1905 he won the Nobel Prize for his tuberculosis work.

In 1947, this acid-fast property that enabled Koch to solve the puzzle of TB came quickly to mind when I found a strange, acid-fast organism present in all the cancers of man and animals I studied. It was, and is, *pleomorphic,* meaning it has many forms during its life cycle, many of which only vaguely, if at all, resemble any other stage. This phenomenon is much the same as the human being's pleomorphic nature—we are zygotes; fetuses; suckling babes; toddlers; teenagers; strong adults; gray and wrinkled seniors.

Until this time, though various kinds of cancer organisms had been observed and described by researchers, the universal property of acid-fastness was not known. I was the first to discover this property, and I immediately began applying this new knowledge to the study of the cause of cancer. If this agent, so obviously related to the TB and leprosy bacilli, was acid-fast, would it cause cancer when injected into laboratory animals? And if so, could the disease itself be treated *with* this bacillus? In other words, could we develop a vaccine from the bacillus; could we *immunize* against cancer using this acid-fast microbe? Further research convinced me that the answer was yes, and from then on my entire future was devoted to proving it. But the story started much earlier.

I was graduated from New York University–Bellevue Medical College in 1936, one of only four women doctors in my class. Previously, I had earned a B.A. in English, history and economics from Vassar. However, the influence of my father, Dr. H. W. Wuerthele, who was one of the early members of the American College of Physicians, and my granduncle, Dr. Joseph Benninghof, a surgeon, had given me an interest in medicine.

Soon after graduating from medical school, I met Dr. Jack Goldberg, commissioner of hospitals, and complained that a woman had never been appointed as a resident or a chief intern at a New York hospital. Ten days later, I was called to his office and informed that I was to become New York City's first woman resident physician. While I was elated, the position wasn't *exactly* what I had in mind—I was to be in charge of the prison ward for venereally infected prostitutes. However, I accepted the job, thinking I would at least clear the way for future women residents, and found it to be one of the most rewarding experiences of my life. My preconceived notions of the prostitute underwent rapid reevaluation, and I developed great compassion for these women, often diseased and discarded by society.

The prison portion of the hospital was located behind a high wall in a compound that also included the infectious disease units of the city hospital. When I attended grand rounds with the other doctors, I had the opportunity to observe several other infectious diseases, especially tuberculosis and leprosy, of which there were many cases in New York City at the time. I began reading all the material I could find about these two related infectious diseases.

Several years later in 1947, when I was a school physician in Newark, New Jersey, one of the school nurses asked if I would look at her hands. She had been diagnosed as having Raynaud's syndrome, a disease in which the ends of the fingers become ulcerated. I noticed that her fingers appeared pinched and became blue after only mild exposure to cold. There were also areas of hypersensitivity along the nerves of her arms and legs. Upon closer examination I found a leprosylike perforation in her septum, the dividing cartilage of the nose. In addition, there were areas of hardness and insensitivity on her skin. My own diagnosis was that she not only had Raynaud's syndrome, but also scleroderma. This disorder not only exhibits hardening of the skin but can involve all of the body's systems and is fatal in a few years if vital organs are affected.

Enlisting the help of my friends Dr. Eva Brodkin, a dermatologist, and Dr. Camille Mermod, a pathologist, I decided to make a full-scale investigation of scleroderma. We made smears from the nurse's nose and finger ulcers and stained them with the acid-fast dyes. To my gratified surprise, numerous organisms of the acid-fast type were visible on the slides. We then obtained surgically aseptic specimens of similar affected lesions and, deep within the body tissues, just as in leprosy, we found the red-dye-retaining microbes. The next step was to make pure cultures of the organisms and inject them into chicks and guinea pigs. Most of the animals became diseased—almost all the chicks died, and the guinea pigs developed hard areas of the skin, similar to scleroderma, and some appeared cancerous. Since the incidence of cancer in guinea pigs is only one in 500,000, this observation took on great significance.

At this point I reasoned that perhaps scleroderma was a kind of slow cancer. I decided to begin examining cancer tissues with the same method, using the acid-fast Ziehl-Neelsen stain. In the meantime, we published the original scleroderma papers concerning the sclerobacillus microorganism. (This work was later confirmed by Del Motte and Van der Mieren at the Pasteur Institute in Brussels in 1953, and in 1971 Dr. Allan Cantwell, a dermatologist at Kaiser-Permanente in Los Angeles, independently found the same microorganism and published his work in the *Archives of Dermatology*.)

Upon examining all kinds of cancerous tissues obtained directly from operating rooms (to insure sterility and absolute freshness), I found that a similar microorganism was present in all of them. I enlisted the assistance of a well-known tissue sectionist in Verona, New Jersey, Dr. Roy M. Allen, and we were again able to demonstrate the presence of acid-fast microbes in the cancerous cells. I was delighted that my concept of the parasitization of the cancer cells by these organisms was verified by someone of such repute. Then Dr. S. J. Rose of St. Michael's Hospital in Newark provided me with a series of unlabeled tissue material, and in every case I was able to pick out the cancerous tissue from healthy tissue by the presence or absence of this microorganism. Both Dr. Allen and Dr. Rose joined me in presenting a paper in August 1948 before the New York Microscopial Society, entitled "Microorganisms Associated with Neoplasms."

When I first conceived of the infectious nature of all cancers, I realized that the predominant thought at the time (and even today) was that cancer is caused by a virus. At that time I thought the micoorganism would probably fall into the group of organisms

I was working with, since the *P. Cryptocides* has filterable (i.e., extremely small) forms that are similar to viruses. Electron microscope studies further verified this concept, and we included photomicrographs in that early paper that showed that the acid-fast microorganisms were present in all forms of human cancer.

At this time I learned of the work of Dr. Eleanor Alexander-Jackson of Cornell University, who had succeeded in demonstrating that the tubercle bacillus undergoes many changes in morphology (size and shape). We formed an association in which she worked with the tubercle and lepra bacilli and I with the *P. Cryptocides*. I was intrigued with the idea that a bacterium could be so wildly pleomorphic, even existing in a form that didn't resemble a bacterium at all. At the time, whether an organism passed through a special filter or not determined whether it was defined as a virus or a bacillus. Viruses, extremely small, passed through; bacilli didn't. Naturally, then, when I started referring to my cancer-causing microbe as a bacillus, related to the tubercle and lepra bacilli, I was not believed.

With Dr. Alexander-Jackson I insisted that various experts hear us out. She was working at Dr. Wilson Smillie's laboratory at Cornell. When Dr. Alexander-Jackson and I explained that we were growing an organism from scleroderma, and that we were convinced there were similar organisms in other collagen diseases, he was about ready to toss Dr. Alexander-Jackson and her strange colleague out the door. However, one of his physicians challenged us with forty blood samples, of which some had been taken from patients with collagen diseases. We soon brought him a 100 percent accurate selection of the twenty-two samples that were infected. This softened Dr. Smillie, and he began to tolerate our work. But when Dr. Alexander-Jackson expressed concern over the future of her work with the tubercle and lepra bacilli in Dr. Smillie's lab, I agreed to stop cluttering up the lab and stay away from Cornell. I then built a laboratory in the basement of my home in New Jersey.

The next major event was in 1949, my formal affiliation with a major university. I had been working with Abbott Laboratories products in developing some of the materials for my scleroderma work. Since we were achieving some remissions in our patients, the Abbott people said they would give me a research grant, but I'd need a university connection.

Due to state antivivisection laws at the time, there were no medical schools in New Jersey. However, Rutgers University, in New Brunswick, had numerous branches around the state, and when Dr. Royal Schaaf, president of Newark Presbyterian Hospital, said he would give me the old nurses' residence next door for a laboratory if I could get Rutgers' affiliation, I saw my chance for the grant. I met with Dr. James Allison, director of the Bureau of Biological Research at Rutgers. He had been very much interested in my work and the confirmation I had received from various associates, and was most knowledgeable and cooperative. On June 2, 1949, I was named head of the new Rutgers-Presbyterian Hospital Laboratory for the Study of Proliferative Diseases, Bureau of Biological Research, Rutgers University. My grant was on its way.

The nurses' residence wasn't much to work with. It resembled an old Victorian brownstone and needed a lot of rehabilitation. Rutgers seemed to think that if we rehabilitated the building, we would be able to attract still more grants. To make a long story short, we raised funds through the gracious help of a local, extremely zealous woman, who induced the local labor unions to turn the nurses' residence into a clean, efficient laboratory.

As a result of the rehabilitation, we applied for a number of substantial grants; these financed our work for the next three years. We received grants from the American Cancer Society, the Damon Runyon Fund, the Rosenwald Foundation, *Reader's Digest*, Charles Pfizer and Company, Lederle Laboratories, the Abbott Company, and many private individuals.

The next few years at Rutgers were to be the most significant period of my work in cancer research. Our research team was enthusiastic that our work would prove once and for all that the P. *Cryptocides* microbe was the cause of cancer and that a vaccine could be made to defend against it.

5

THE DISCOVERY OF THE CANCER MICROBE, II

RUTGERS UNIVERSITY

Now that we had the necessary facilities at Newark, under Rutgers University auspices, we were able to expand through the acquisition of several grants. I became an associate professor in the Bureau of Biological Research and proceeded to build my research team. Dr. Eleanor Alexander-Jackson was my first choice. She had decided to research cancer infection for herself and had obtained fresh tumors under sterile conditions from Memorial Hospital at Cornell. After studying the cultures from these tumors she confirmed that the specific organism, *P. Cryptocides*, was present in all the tumors she examined. It wasn't hard after that to convince Eleanor to leave Cornell and join us at Rutgers. She commuted daily from New York to work in our lab as our bacteriologist. The rest of the team consisted of Dr. Roy Allen, our histologist, who kept himself and an assistant busy preparing tissue sections of material; Dr. Lawrence W. Smith, our pathologist; Joseph Patti, an experienced animal-tumor expert from a distinguished institute in New York; Marilyn Clark, a tissue culturist; and Andrew Steciuw, who cared for the experimental animals.

In the five years from 1949 to 1953 a great deal was accomplished. I was assigned a number of hospital beds to which I could bring cancer patients for study, and we had access to fresh cancer material from the hospital operating rooms. We had the full cooperation of the Presbyterian Hospital under Dr. Royal Schaaf, and of Rutgers University itself under Dr. James Allison. We collected and studied all the obtainable animal tumors believed to be infectious in nature and supposedly caused by a virus. They were the Rous, Walker, Sprague-Dawley, Shope, and Sarcoma-180 tumors, plus various types of fowl neoplasia. From these we made cultures, bacterial isolates, that we compared with cultures derived from many types of fresh, uncontaminated human tumors from the blood and other body fluids of patients with advanced cancer. As anticipated, these cultures had a great similarity to one another. There were some variations as to size and some differences in the kind of media or material in which they would grow. Certain strains fermented one kind of sugar, some others. Some could live with little or no oxygen, some required more. Dr. Alexander-Jackson studied various peptones, or protein fractions, until she found those that were best for producing good growth of the organisms in test tubes. I worked with making a medium from chick embryos.

All of these culture studies supported the growth of the organism well. Over and over our organisms *Progenitor Cryptocides* were acid-fast and highly pleomorphic in their growth pattern. They stained with the Ziehl-Neelsen stain in the same way as did the tubercle bacillus, which causes tuberculosis. The bacteriologists at Rutgers University were satisfied that we had pure cultures free of contamination from other bacteria. (Contamination is always the most important problem in the isolation of microorganisms. Contaminants are present everywhere. Usually, they are harmless bacteria from the air or soil, or from humans or animals. The danger is that they may simulate the real culprits, the pathogens, the disease producers. No laboratory is ever free of them. In fact, it was the contamination of Sir Alexander Fleming's cultures by the penicillium mold that led to his famous discovery of pencillin.)

Our cultures were scrutinized repeatedly. Strains of the P.C. were sent to many laboratories for identification; none could really classify them. They were something unknown. They had many forms, but they always evolved into the same microbe no matter how often they were cultured. The P.C.s resembled the mycobacteria more than anything else. (The tubercle bacillus is a mycobacterium or fungoid bacillus.) When our advisers at Rutgers felt that we had pure, uncontaminated cultures, we were ready to follow Koch's law, or postulates. Koch's law is the accepted foolproof method of proving the cause of a disease. Koch's postulates are:

1. The microorganism must be present in every case of the disease.
2. It must be possible to cultivate the microorganism outside the host (i.e., animal) in some artificial medium.
3. The inoculation of this culture must produce the disease in a susceptible animal.
4. The microorganism must then be reobtained from these inoculated animals and cultured again.

We were able to fulfill Koch's postulates. The culmination of this work was published in the *American Journal of Medical Sciences* in December 1950. It was entitled "Cultural Properties and Pathogenicity of Certain Microorganisms Obtained from Various Proliferative and Neoplastic Diseases." There were four authors besides myself and Dr. Alexander-Jackson. They were Dr. John A. Anderson, head of the Department of Bacteriology at Rutgers; Dr. James Hillier, developer of the electron microscope and head of electron microscopy at the RCA Victor Laboratories in Princeton, New Jersey; Dr. Roy M. Allen, noted histologist; and Dr. Lawrence W. Smith, author of a well-known pathology textbook used in medical colleges.

This paper was the culmination of several years of effort, starting with my early scleroderma work in the mid-1940s. It required three months of scrutiny by the Rutgers group headed by Drs. James Allison and John Anderson before passing their rigid requirements for publication. It stands today as a milestone on the infectious nature of cancer.

The paper described how pure cultures were obtained from the various cancers of both human beings and animals. These were then injected into animals capable of being infected. Gradually, diseased areas developed that resembled those from which the cultures were obtained. Then pure cultures were reisolated from the infected animals. Koch's postulates were fulfilled to the satisfaction of our entire group and to that of our biology superiors at Rutgers.

The next step was to prove that the cancerous growth itself was not the whole disease. For more than one hundred years people like Rudolf Virchow thought that cancer cells themselves were parasites within the body. He did not understand that the small coccuslike granules he saw dividing in the cancers were not the development of daughter cells within mother cells, but that instead they represented the true intracellular parasite that was the causative agent. In his book, *The Savage Cell*, Patrick McGrady defines cancer as "a savage cell which somehow evades the laws of the body, corrupts the forces which normally protect the body, invades the well-ordered society of cells that surrounds it, colonizes distant areas, and as a finale to its cannibalistic orgy of flesh consuming flesh, commits suicide by destroying its host." This is a picturesque and dramatic description of the cancer cell, but it's not entirely true. The whole truth may be that the parasite within the cancer transforms the normal cell into a sick cell that cannot mature by normal cell growth processes. In other words, the tumor itself is *not* the disease.

No one today believes that the pleomorphic lesions of syphilis, which can appear anywhere in the body of an untreated person, constitute the disease itself. Volumes have been written about the cause and cure of syphilis. The effects of the disease, like cancer, have reached into every corner of the civilized world. Mighty kings fathered syphilitic weaklings. The stigma bridging the generations became the basis for Ibsen's famous play *Ghosts*.

Then in 1905 Fritz Schaudinn found the cause, the spirochete *Treponema Pallidum*. The microbe causes the disease. The search for the cure began: injections of arsenicals, mercury, and bismuth, to name but a few. These were often dangerous and not always effective. Such treatments gave rise to the famous saying, "One night with Venus and ten years with Mercury." Then in 1928 came Sir Alexander Fleming's great discovery. We can now say Syphilis: Penicillin. All is said in two words.

Dr. Francisco Duran-Reynals, in the years from 1940 to 1956, showed that the Rous "virus," or tumor agent, could cause acute and lethal hemorrhagic disease when given in large amounts, but smaller amounts could lead to a lesser reaction resulting in cancer. With a still further repression of the tumor infectious agent, chronic, interstitial disease similar to arthritis and heart disease would appear in the experimental animals. Dr. Duran-Reynals also proved that the Rous "virus," or tumor agent, can cross species barriers and infect ducks and turkeys; and that filtrates—that is, filtered material from tumor tissue, not the cells themselves—can transmit Rous sarcoma to guinea pigs, rabbits, and marmosets.

Our paper, "Cultural Properties and Pathogenicity of Certain Microorganisms Obtained from Various Proliferative and Neoplastic Diseases," proved that the tumor was *not* the disease. It was the *P. Cryptocides* that caused the disease in the animals and so fulfilled Koch's postulates. In 1948 we were years ahead of others in showing that the Rous tumor agent was not a virus but a pleomorphic bacterium. It was the *P. Cryptocides* microbe. As in Duran-Reynals's work, the tumors were only a part of the resultant disease. In addition to tumors, there were cheesy lesions or areas resembling tuberculosis, which could invade any one of the essential organs such as the liver, kidney, heart, or lung. These organs might show changes in the connective tissue, called collagen, that could lead to degeneration as seen in the chronic human degenerative diseases. So it was concluded that these microorganisms, *P. Cryptocides*, could not only cause cancer but a number of other ailments that afflict man. The infectious nature of arthritis, of some kinds of heart, liver, and kidney impairment, and most recently diabetes, has been proposed. Many medical researchers admit that the patterns of these diseases point to their latent infectious nature, but no one has come forth with an antigen or actual causative agent. It is these filterable forms of the *P. Cryptocides* that have been described as C-particles, mycoplasma, or viruses by other research workers. I propose that certain strains of the *Progenitor* group are the culprits.

Before the theory that the filterable form of the *Progenitor* group was equivalent to the so-called tumor-viruses could be proven, it was necessary for us to spend many months working with Dr. James Hillier of the RCA Victor Laboratories in Princeton. There the bacterial cultures isolated from human and animal tumors were passed through filters that permitted passage only of so-called true viruses. These filtrates contained minute forms of life which then regrew to become bacterial cultures. This work proved conclusively that the Rous agent was not a virus. Peyton Rous did not call his tumor filtrates viruses but "filterable microbial agents," or "tumor agents." A true virus has been defined as a submicroscopic infectious unit that lives only in the presence of living cells and cannot exist even momentarily outside of them. But Rous's "tumor agents" could be dried, stored on a shelf at room temperature for years, and when mixed with saline could then be reactivated to initiate fresh tumors. Therefore, these "tumor agents" are definitely *not* viruses. A great deal of time and effort has been spent in trying to find a virus implicated in any form of human cancer. *None has been proven.* However, I was proposing that the filterable forms of *P. Cryptocides*, which are of virus size, are the causative agents in human and animal cancers, and that, like the Rous "tumor agents," they are transmissible from one animal to another. There was some criticism in those days stating that mice often developed cancer spontaneously and that therefore it would be better to work with other animals as well. However, in all research the results are judged by the comparison of the treated animal with the untreated controls, so that even if there are cancers in the untreated, there is a significant differential. The need for genetically controlled mice led to the development of certain inbred strains having predictable sites and numbers of tumors. We also used these strains as well as guinea pigs, which have a natural immunity and are resistant to cancer. Only 1 guinea pig in 500,000 develops cancer spontaneously. We were able to produce tumors in an amazing 25 percent.

It was while working with guinea pigs that my suspicions as to the method of transmissibility of tumors were confirmed. Due to an error, the infected guinea pigs were housed in cages at the top of the racks while the healthy, uninoculated controls, instead of being housed on different racks, were placed in cages underneath. To our surprise, the control animals also developed cancer. On careful inspection we found that droppings from the top cages sometimes fell into the drinking water and food of the guinea pigs below. From that time on we kept the controls in separate rooms. Our animal man changed his gown, cap, mask, and gloves before going from one area to the other. The guinea pig controls thereafter stopped developing cancer. My convictions about transmissibility of cancer grew.

We tried to ascertain the effect of our cancer cultures on living tissue cultures, that is, on uncontaminated, totally clean tissue in test tubes (*in vitro*). These tissues were living cells nourished by various types of nutritive material, some artificial and some taken from serum of chickens and calves. We found that under the influence of the microbes the tissue cultures showed marked changes, such as degeneration and destruction of cells with abnormal cell division. However, I suspected that since the embryo fluids used for nourishing the tissue cultures came from chicks, they might contain the cancer agent. This proved to be the case, since many chickens and their eggs have the pathogenic form of the cancer microbe. (See Chapter Nine). Thereafter, whenever "spontaneous" conversion of a tissue culture to the cancerous state was described in the literature, I would be most skeptical as to the cause. Again, it was the difference between the infected and the uninfected tissue cultures that was significant in short-term studies. (Later, Dr. Irene Corey Diller of the Department of Pathology, the Institute for Cancer Research, and Dr. William F. Diller, Department of Biology, University of Pennsylvania, were to perform some excellent experiments with cancer cultures in living tissue, which confirmed the conversion of normal cells to abnormal cells by the inoculation of the *P. Cryptocides* cancer microbes into the tissue culture of cells.)

At times the work that Dr. Alexander-Jackson and I did was sad and unpleasant. It seemed to me that it was important to study one kind of human cancer thoroughly. We decided that the cancer of the human breast would be the most suitable since the cancers usually were enclosed within the breast and not subject to contamination from the bowel or adjacent structures. Also, they are a common type of cancer and not too difficult to obtain. I collected thirty breasts that had been removed for cancer from the operating rooms. They were fresh from the surgeon's knife, obtained directly after the pathologist had taken specimens for sectioning. They were, of course, kept sterile. They were brought back to the laboratory, where we dissected the cancers and the glands from under the arm, or axilla. We numbered the specimens, cultured not only the tumors but the glands as well, and compared them with the pathologists' reports. In *all* of the cases where we could obtain blood samples, we grew positive cultures from the blood. Also, even when the pathologist reported that the underarm glands were negative for tumor cells, *the cancer organisms developed from them when cultured. These results showed that cancer is not a localized, but a generalized (systemic), disease.*

Later, in March 1953, when our group was invited to present papers at the Sixth International Congress of Microbiology in Rome, I invited Dr. George Clark, a pathologist, to attend with us.

Dr. Clark was an exceptionally well-trained pathologist from Scranton, Penn., who had reported, in 1920, on the successful culturing of Glover's cancer organism and the development of metastasizing tumors in animals brought on by injections of human malignancy cultures. What he had called the "Glover organism" in 1920 was undoubtedly the same as our organism. However, most of the work of Dr. Thomas Glover's, a Canadian, was unpublished. When Dr. Clark and his associates were invited to Washington, D.C., to repeat the experiments, under the supervision of Dr. George W. McCoy, Director of Public Health, they remained there for eight years and their work, too, was never published. To this day, I don't know why.

At the Congress, Dr. Clark presented a scholarly paper. It was gratifying that after many sacrifices, tribulations and the suppression of his work, I could give Dr. Clark the opportunity to present it. Prior to the Rome meeting we all met in Scranton to compare notes with earlier workers such as Drs. Jacob Engle, H. B. Leffler, and M. J. Scott. We also raised sufficient funds to bring Dr. Franz Gerlach from Germany to be honored in Scranton at a "Gerlach Day" celebration. He had devoted much of his life in Vienna to the study of the cancer parasite, which he called a "micromycete." (It has always been my conviction that there is no place in research for jealousy or destructive competition. How often has a truth been suppressed or recognition delayed because selfish peers would not recognize the merit of a fellow worker!)

While Dr. Clark was visiting, he reported that Glover had been able to produce antibodies and antiserum in sheep and horses that were beneficial in the treatment of human cancer. Using Glover's method, we decided to try to reproduce his work by immunizing sheep with an attenuated, or weakened, culture. Dr. Harriette Vera, chief bacteriologist at and one of the owners of the Baltimore Biological Laboratories, who had done much of the confirmatory work with our cultures, sent us a generous contribution which enabled us to perform this experiment.

First we needed an area in which to keep our experimental animals. I had a patient in Nutley, N.J., who owned a dairy farm. He agreed to rent us a small remote pasture. Then I purchased a flock of twenty sheep and engaged a state veterinarian to assist us. He examined the sheep and found them free of disease. We attenuated some of the stock vaccines we had on hand, such as cultures from human breast cancer; from a sarcoma of a young boy; from a human leukemia; from the Rous chicken tumor; from arthritis; and from fowl leukosis. We injected two sheep with each strain. After about four weeks the veterinarian reported that some of the sheep were getting sick. We examined the sheep weekly and provided the veterinarian with the attenuated vaccines from the cancer cultures, which he used for immunization. Several ewes aborted their young. The fetuses were macerated. Some of the sheep developed very swollen painful joints and could scarcely graze. Others looked sickly and got thin. We realized that the organisms in our vaccines were still alive, and not dead as they should have been to make a weak enough vaccine for immunization without actually giving the sheep a disease. In other words, we had not fully immunized the sheep, but had given them the disease with the living organisms in our vaccine. We asked the veterinarian to bleed the sheep in order to assay their serum for antibodies. We received the sterile sera, but the sheep had to be destroyed and carried away for incineration. I was so concerned for fear the soil of the farmer's pasture might be contaminated that I sent for the Nutley Fire Department to burn over the entire field with all the fodder that had been given to the sheep. Nature would have to do the rest in sterilizing the soil.

Although the sheep had to be destroyed, we learned a great deal from that experiment. We learned that the chicken vaccine agglutinated in high dilution with the cultures from the boy's sarcoma; that breast cancer serum reacted with the human leukemia isolates; and the Rous sarcoma serum reacted with all of the cultures. This meant that the human cultures cross-reacted with one another strongly and also cross-reacted with the animal serum samples, showing that tumors are not specific to certain organs or species. *In other words, the tumors could be transmitted from one type of tissue to another, from one kind of animal to another.*

We next turned our attention to fowl leukosis, a cancerous disease that was killing many fowl on the poultry farms of New

Jersey. We went to Verona, N.J. to interview a chicken rancher we knew. He said that he was losing about 25 percent of his chickens to fowl leukosis. We asked him if we might have some of his sick birds. He handed us three chickens that could no longer stand up. We took them to the laboratory, and in a short time they were dead. We then took samples of their hearts' blood, which grew into the same kind of cultures as those derived from all of our other tumors.

We decided that this time we would completely inactivate the cultures. That is, we would be sure that they were killed before we used them to produce antibodies, this time in rabbits. We thoroughly immunized two sets of rabbits, one set with a tissue vaccine made from the tumor, and the other one with a bacterial vaccine made from the cultured microbes, both from the chickens. We bled the rabbits and refrigerated the serum. Then we went back to the Verona rancher and asked him for six more dying chickens. All six were so weak, they could no longer stand. Their heads fell over, and they lay on their sides twitching from time to time, their beaks open.

We separated the chickens into three groups of two. The two we did not treat died before morning. Two were treated with the rabbit antiserum produced by tumor cell vaccine, and two were treated with the rabbit antiserum from the bacterial vaccine. We then watched them carefully. In just a few hours all four got up on their legs and were able to drink water. We treated them for several days with all the rabbit serum we had. All four recovered completely. The ones that received the tissue vaccine recovered more slowly and were somewhat stunted in growth. The two chickens treated with the bacterial vaccine became very vigorous, full-fleshed roosters. After several months we destroyed the stunted birds. But they were tumor-free! The other two roosters we kept for one year, and they remained perfectly clear of any tumors.

One day while I was making rounds in the hospital, one of the patients remarked, "You'd think we were out in the country instead of in the middle of the city. Every morning at daylight a couple of roosters crow so loudly we're all awakened out of a sound sleep. I wonder who's keeping them in the neighborhood?" I took the hint. When one of the janitors remarked that they were mighty fine looking birds and would make a nice dinner for someone, we gave them to him for his Christmas dinner. We knew that he could never find such beautiful birds anywhere on the market. Whatever fowl he might have bought for dinner would have been infected with cancer, but our rabbit antiserum had cured the cancer in our chickens. Most important, it was the antiserum produced in the rabbits with the pure bacterial *P. Cryptocides* cultures that was the curative agent.

6

THE DISCOVERY OF THE CANCER MICROBE, III

A BETRAYAL CLOSES THE LAB

ALTHOUGH THE RESEARCH WORK we were doing was confirmed by many corroborative workers, there continued to be considerable friction between our group and the groups that directed their efforts not toward the microbic cause of cancer but toward the cancer cell itself. Their theory was that, if you could destroy the cancer cell, you could conquer the disease. This was essentially the theory that Rudolf Virchow had proposed so many years ago: The cancer cell acts parasitically upon the body, and one has only to destroy it to cure the cancer. This is a completely erroneous principle that still persists.

How many patients over the years have asked in complete bewilderment, "Doctor, why has my cancer come back? They said they got it all, and now it is spread all over." The complete removal of the cancer, as explained in Chapter Three, may have some influence upon the course of the disease, but is not the determining factor in the survival of the patient. *Immunity is the answer.* If a patient's immune system is not at maximum strength, the smallest tumor completely removed will not prevent other tumors from arising in other parts of the body.

At the time of our Rutgers discoveries many of the large research centers, such as the Memorial Sloan-Kettering Cancer Center in New York City, were dedicated largely to finding a chemical or group of chemicals that would destroy the cancer *cell*. Dr. Cornelius P. Rhoads, then director of Sloan-Kettering, would brook no competition or interference from anyone who disagreed with his concepts along this line. He considered us along with our collaborators an upstart group. He was often heard to say, "When the cause and cure of cancer is found, I will find it." He died a disappointed man.

It is always amazing how fallacious conclusions of researchers associated with large, heavily endowed institutions can sway the minds of scientists and physicians all over the world, blinding them to the scientific truth. This was the case with Cornelius Rhoads. The Memorial Sloan-Kettering Hospital was heavily endowed with millions of dollars from private industrial giants, and Rhoads wielded his authority like a heavy club. He himself was less a scientist than a promoter and a politician determined to perpetuate the powerful cancer interests vested in him and his institution.

Dr. Rhoads was committed to chemotherapy, and well he might have been since he was head of chemical warfare during most of World War II. He tried to turn chemical warfare against the cancer cell within the human body. His great mistake was that he believed the cancer *cell* to be the causative agent of the disease, and not the parasite contained *within* the cell. To unleash the horrors of chemical warfare and the atomic bomb in the form of chemotherapy and cobalt radiation against the helpless victims of a microbic disease is illogical. Further, Dr. Rhoads was not content to limit his theories to his own institution but was determined to dictate the research policies of the entire country. At one point he almost succeeded in destroying the basic biological research at the Institute for Cancer Research in Philadelphia and turning the institute into a subservient satellite. Fortunately, he failed.

About 1950, Dr. Irene Diller of the Institute for Cancer Research in Philadelphia attempted to set up a symposium at the

New York Academy of Sciences in order to present a number of papers concerning our work on the microbic infectious nature of cancer. The meeting was killed by Dr. Rhoads. All he needed was something to discredit one of us. Dr. Diller had accepted from a commercial company several ultraviolet sterilizing lights for her laboratory. There were no strings attached. However, Dr. Rhoads used her acceptance of this gift to state that she had "commercialized" her work and therefore was not eligible to sponsor a symposium. (It was to be 1969 before we finally held our symposium at the New York Academy of Sciences.)

One day in 1951, Eleanor said to me, "I hate to bring this up but I have a lump in my left breast." She came over to my office, where I examined her. She certainly did have a sizable hard mass in the inner upper quadrant of her left breast. There was no question in my mind as to what it was. Dr. Frank Adair at the Memorial Center arranged for her to have surgery. The tumor was malignant, and Eleanor underwent a radical mastectomy. Her father, Dr. Jerome Alexander, and I stood by anxiously during the surgery. While we were waiting, I was summoned over the loudspeaker to Dr. Rhoads' office. I went there immediately. Dr. Rhoads motioned me to a chair in his large, luxurious office overlooking East Sixty-eighth Street. He was an imposing man, tall and quite handsome.

"You people can help us a great deal with our research," he said. I thought to myself, how ironic—now that Eleanor herself is afflicted with the disease, he has softened and will be more cooperative in our work. Then he continued, "We have been looking for a tumor such as she has. One on the inner side of the breast where the glands draining the tumor lie within the mediastinum. (This is an area between the lungs where the great vessels come from the heart. It is fairly inaccessible.) We would like to have someone to try out a new surgical technique. She could be the first one to have her sternum (the breast bone) split, permitting us to do a dissection around the heart and great vessels to remove the glands there. We have not been able to get permission from anyone for this surgery. She would be performing a great service in permitting us to do this, as it would be an experiment to see how it would affect a patient and to determine the length of time she might survive."

I was speechless. He wanted me to talk Eleanor into having the experimental operation! This man had been discrediting our research at every turn, and now he was talking about my dear friend and loyal colleague as if she were an experimental animal. I was infuriated. "Not on your life!" I told him. "That is a cruel and disfiguring operation. Her body could be so shocked that she might not even withstand the operation. She didn't even *need* a radical, since her glands did not drain toward the axilla. I will oppose the idea with every ounce of persuasion I have." I left the room with tears in my eyes. He had not called me to his office to commiserate, to sympathize, or to help, but only to ask that Eleanor be sacrificed on his altar of research.

Eleanor came through the surgery splendidly. The next day when I told her what Dr. Rhoads wanted me to suggest to her, she was most indignant. "We should stand by what we believe," she said sternly. "I won't have any cobalt treatments or any further surgery. I'll watch my diet and take our vaccines." This she did. It is now more than thirty years since that fateful day. Eleanor says she has never had the slightest evidence of a return of her tumor. She recuperated rapidly and was back at the laboratory in a short time. Eleanor has always been a woman of great stamina and determination. Her daily trips to the Newark laboratory in the freezing cold or the blazing heat were feats of endurance. It took at least one and a half hours from her apartment on Riverside Drive to the laboratory. She was always cheerful, eager, and interested in our work. Every step of the way was a great adventure that we shared. Sometimes we differed and quarreled; sometimes one felt put upon by the other, but reason always shone through. Our friendship has continued all these years. Though we are very different people, we have been held together by our interest in the microbial nature of cancer, and each by faith in the integrity and good judgment of the other. My admiration for her father, Dr. Jerome Alexander, was profound. He was not only a brilliant chemist but a great humanitarian.

During the Rutgers years we made every effort to coordinate

our work with related microbial procedures. We visited a number of scientists who were interested in our approach to the cancer problem. In 1949, before Rutgers would consider accepting my projects under their auspices, Dr. James Allison and I had traveled to Philadelphia to meet Dr. Margaret Lewis at the Wistar Institute. She and her husband had spent a lifetime of research in the microbiology of cancer. A great deal of their work had been done with the rat, and Dr. Lewis had stored paraffin blocks of experimental rat cancer in her laboratory. After we had conversed for some time, I said, "You can give me any one of those tumor blocks, and I will demonstrate with proper staining the causative organisms in the sections." Dr. Lewis gave us a block of tissue from the shelf at random. Even without the corroboration of the stained slides, she told Dr. Allison that she thought my work should be associated with Rutgers University. I turned the tissue block over to Dr. Roy Allen, who prepared the sections with our special stains. As expected, the hidden killer *P. Cryptocides* was revealed throughout the tumor by the acid-fast stain. The stained sections were then sent to Dr. Lewis and Dr. Allison.

After Dr. Eleanor Alexander-Jackson joined our laboratory, we continued to visit various clinics and research centers. I was especially interested in meeting with Dr. Elise L'Esperance of what was then the Strang Memorial Cancer Detection Clinic in New York City. Not only had she founded the world's first cancer detection clinic, but she also had worked on the microbic theory of cancer. When I was a student at Bellevue Medical College, a pathology professor had said rather disparagingly, "There is a woman pathologist at Cornell who thinks Hodgkin's disease (a form of glandular cancer) is caused by avian tuberculosis. She has published a report on this, but no one has confirmed her findings." As I looked into the microscope at the slides of Hodgkin's disease I could not help comparing them with the slides I had seen of tuberculosis. In Hodgkin's disease, the large multinucleated giant cells are called Reed-Sternberg cells. They are similar to the giant cells of tuberculosis. In tuberculosis these cells form and engulf the tubercle bacilli. I stored away the thought that Dr. L'Esperance was probably right, but she would have a difficult time gaining acceptance. Years later, after I had made my initial observations of the acid-fast tuberculosislike forms in scleroderma, followed by observations of the same forms in all cancers including Hodgkin's disease, I remembered Dr. L'Esperance.

Sometime in 1950, while we were at the Newark laboratory, I phoned Dr. L'Esperance. She said she would be glad to see Eleanor and me and asked us to meet her at the Strang Memorial Cancer Detection Clinic. I knew something about the founding of the Strang center and was most anxious to see the clinic. Dr. L'Esperance had been very active for years at the New York Women's Infirmary, where she established her first cancer detection center. She and her sister, May Strang, were nieces and heirs of Chauncey Depew, president of the New York Central Railroad and a famous after-dinner speaker. After his death the two women inherited a great deal of money. They founded the Kate Depew Strang Memorial Cancer Detection Clinic in memory of their mother, who had died of cancer. It was the first clinic of its kind in the world.

We met with Dr. L'Esperance, who greeted us cordially and showed us around the clinic. In the year after the clinic was started only forty-one patients went through. In its last eight months, in 1950, more than two thousand were screened. During this time Dr. L'Esperance had established the validity and utility of the work of Dr. George N. Papanicolaou, M.D., Ph.D., who became known as the father of modern cytology because of his outstanding contribution in the field of exfoliative cytology. We met him that day in his laboratory, where he showed us some of his work. Today, it is thanks to his research that women are having their Pap smears regularly, "Pap" being the shortened form of his last name. In a Pap smear the body cells that are cast off from the uterus, cervix, and vagina are scraped from the cervix, placed on a slide, and stained. Not only is the presence of cancer cells detected, but the amount of the body's estrogen is indicated by the size and shape of each cell's nucleus in relation to the cytoplasm. This test is also useful for determining the stage of menopause in women. Unfortunately, when the smear for cancer is positive, the cancer is already there. However, this test does permit early detection of some kinds of cancer of the female reproductive organs. The same method of cell determination is now applied to a number of other sites, such as lung and stomach. Until Dr. L'Esperance demonstrated the usefulness of the Pap smear at her cancer detection clinics, Dr. Papanicolaou's work was not accepted in medical circles.

It was a thrill for me to tell Dr. L'Esperance that I had found acid-fast organisms in all the tumors I had examined, and they seemed to be similar to the ones she had observed in Hodgkin's disease. I explained that we had cultured them, and that they were producing tumors in experimental animals. Dr. L'Esperance said she hoped that we would have better success than she had had when she was doing her early work with Hodgkin's disease. She told us how she had isolated the acid-fast organisms from the glands of patients, made a culture, and then inoculated the organisms into guinea pigs. She reproduced the lesions and cultured the organisms again, fulfilling Koch's postulates. When she showed the animal tissues to Dr. James Ewing, the famous pathologist at the Cornell Medical Center, he confirmed the fact that the tissues were Hodgkin's disease. When she told him that they were from experimentally inoculated guinea pigs, he then insisted that they were not Hodgkin's disease, that it was impossible to reproduce the disease by cultures. Dr. L'Esperance was disgusted but continued on with her work at the Strang Clinic until the technician she depended upon became ill; she was never able to replace her and retired soon after.

During 1950 we made many trips to Princeton to take our filtered cultures to Dr. James Hillier of the RCA Victor Laboratories for electron microscopy. Dr. Hillier was very exacting in his studies of *P. Cryptocides*. Many of the smaller bodies were beyond the range of the standard microscope and were filterable on the basis of size alone. Repeated electron microscopic studies were made before and after passage through mice of pure microbic strains isolated from patients with cancer and scleroderma, and from chickens infected with the Rous "virus," or tumor agent. The filtered bodies appeared to be the same size as viruses. An electron photograph of the particles seen in mouse leukemia, and a similar one of the microbic structures we isolated in culture, illustrated the fact that the bodies in the mouse tissues and those we cultured are undoubtedly the same agent. We feel that these studies definitely demonstrate that the so-called virus (or the C-particles, or the L-forms, or whatever name is currently in vogue) is the filterable form of this microbe, the hidden killer, *P. Cryptocides.*

We exhibited our electron work at a number of meetings and received great commendation and an award of merit on one occasion. These cancer microbes are so tough and resistant to heat that at our 1953 exhibit at the New York American Medical Association, the microbes stayed alive for five days while being televised by closed circuitry. We were indebted to the RCA Victor people for providing the television setup and an engineer to operate it for an entire week. Visitors could watch the living bugs swimming about through the microscope on television; it was the sensation of the exhibit. The press coverage would have been great, but again the formidable Dr. Rhoads forbade the N.Y.A.M.A. publicity people to interview us. He also threatened to withhold further news releases from the press if they reported on our findings. They were intimidated by him and did not mention our exhibit at all, although there were crowds of people waiting to get into our booth. Again because of politics, we lost yet another chance to bring attention to our work.

We had many other meetings of great interest. We visited Dr. Peyton Rous at the Rockefeller Institute. This future Nobel laureate was very kindly and interested in our work. We told him about growing the Rous agent in artificial media outside of the living cell. He said that he did not think this was unlikely or impossible. (When he received the Nobel Prize for Medicine in 1966 at the age of eighty-seven, it was more than a half century since he had first reported the infectious nature of the chicken tumor, which later bore his name.) We further met with Dr. Richard Shope, also of the Rockefeller Institute, who had identified the infectious agent of a rabbit tumor. On one occasion, at a meeting in Newark, I had the temerity to differ with Dr. Shope on the type of cell in the Rous tumor that would transmit the cancer. Dr. Shope claimed that only the tumor cell could infect fresh chickens. I insisted that this was not true, that any cell of the infected chicken could pass on the cancer, and that it need not be a cancer cell but the *P. Cryptocides* microbe in any seemingly normal cell from the infected host which could do so. In the case of blood, the serum had to be washed away, but the red blood cell itself could transmit the disease as well as any other cell, whether cancerous or not. To me this was and is an extremely important point, because whether a chicken displays a cancerous growth or not, many still contain the cancerous infectious agent within their bodies. *This is the reason it is not advisable for the cancer patient to eat poultry.* Since it is transmissible to the ape, it was obvious to me, at least, that it can be transmitted to a susceptible human being. However, Dr. Shope took issue with me and did not agree but promised to look up the information. In a few days, a generous letter of apology arrived stating that my premise was correct and that he had been misinformed.

We also visited the Lederle Laboratories at Pearl River, where we became acquainted with Paul Little, who was in charge of their antitumor agent screening program. Mr. Little worked largely with the Rous sarcoma. At this point Lederle was excited about antifolic agents, the folic-acid antagonists. Folic acid, a B vitamin, is the component processed by the liver that is essential for the prevention of pernicious anemia, a form of anemia that was considered fatal until the protective effects of liver and, later, folic acid were discovered. At the time we were visiting Lederle Laboratories, it was felt that substances that substituted for and opposed folic acid could destroy tumors. These are called *analogs,* counterfeits of the real vitamin made to "fool" the cancer cell in its requirement for the essential vitamin; the cancer incorporates the counterfeit into the cell and is killed. This is a kind of nutritional Trojan horse. In 1948 Dr. Sidney Farber of Children's Hospital in Boston initiated the era of analogs in cancer research by injecting some children with a drug called aminopterin, after which they showed a remarkable return to health. Unfortunately, the recovery was only temporary; at best a few lived up to a year or two. Aminopterin is still in use today. Farber's minor success touched off a search for analogs, false vitamins, false hormones, and other chemcial agents. However, I was not impressed, because even though chickens previously infected with Rous sarcoma and then given Dr. Farber's analog did not develop tumors, they either died of folic-acid deprivation or of other forms of the Rous disease. I warned Mr. Little that our bacterial cultures of the Rous-infected chickens treated with the folic-acid antagonists showed no diminution in the amount of growth of the causative agent. There were numerous round-table discussions with the staff at Lederle. Although conducted in a congenial atmosphere, the conversations always ended in a draw or stalemate. I couldn't agree with them, and they thought a bacterial culture from a so-called virus-induced tumor, such as Rous sarcoma, was impossible.

On another occasion we went to the Bronx Botanical Gardens to request some cultures of *Bacterium tumefaciens* (*agrobacterium tumefaciens*). Although Erwin Frank Smith discovered *Bacterium tumefaciens* in January 1908, he did not report his production of malignant growth in plants with this microorganism until April 1916 in the *Journal of Cancer Research*. Smith was a noted pathologist in charge of the laboratory of plant pathology for the U.S. Department of Agriculture. He was also a bacteriologist and in 1906, president of the Society of American Bacteriologists. He produced cancers in plants at will by injections of *Bacterium tumefaciens*. In plants these tumors are called *crown galls*. The diseased plants can be seen anywhere in the United States if one just knows what to look for. A number of investigators thought that *Bacterium tumefaciens* could produce cancers in animals and perhaps even in humans. The work of Erwin F. Smith had a profound influence on Dr. Charles Mayo of the famed Mayo Clinic, who reported on October 28, 1925, at an American College of Surgeons meeting:

Down in Washington, in the government laboratories of the Department of Agriculture, Erwin Smith, a very well-known government bacteriologist, is carrying on a most interesting series of experiments on plants. He has rows on rows of plants in which he has been able to transplant cancer, resembling the disease in human beings. So exact are his experiments that he is able to foretell with absolute accuracy just how long it will require the cancerous growth to break out on the plant stock, and more than that, just where it will break out.

At the Bronx Botanical Gardens we were given a tube of the living microbes and admonished not to drop the bottle, as we had enough there to infect half of the state of New York. Needless to say, Eleanor held the bottle very securely while I drove back to the Newark laboratory. We observed the microbes in culture and then injected a living culture into mice. With large doses, the mice died overnight; with small doses they lived longer. Dr. Franz Gerlach, who was at the laboratory at the time, thought that on gross examination the diseased tissues resembled sarcomas. However, we did not pursue this study any further except to note that the culture was pathogenic for mice on injection. We have electron photographs of this culture. The organism appears to be endemic in the soil, but it may also be transmitted by an insect vector. (We had a young peach tree in our yard which appeared healthy and had pretty blossoms in spring. However, several of the peaches that ripened on it had tumorous swellings on them. On staining these tumors we found bacilli. I warned my husband not to eat the peaches but to cut down the tree and to burn it. I have always felt that all trees and vegetation bearing the crown gall should be destroyed by burning and the underlying soil sterilized, if possible.)

Recently an exciting article appeared in *Scientific American,* June 1983—"A Vector for Introducing New Genes into Plants."

It described how a bacterium, *H. tumefaciens*, can insert a piece of its DNA into a healthy plant cell causing a genetic modification in the plant cell causing it to become a cancer cell which multiplies into a full tumor called Crown Gall Tumor. The mechanisms of this transformation are fully explained. No virus is implicated. If a bacterium can transform a healthy cell of a plant into a plant cancer, is it not reasonable to suppose a human bacterium could transform a healthy human cell into a human cancer without any implication of a virus?

There is a marked similarity in the way P. Cryptocides evolves a genome to produce CG in the cell. The major difference is that P.C. is latent in the normal cell and becomes a bacterial revertant producing CG under certain conditions.

Of our many associations, our visits with Drs. Irene and William Diller of Philadelphia were the most rewarding and enjoyable. Dr. Irene Diller, editor of the biological journal *Growth*, was associated with the Institute for Cancer Research at Fox Chase, Philadelphia. She is not only a famous research scientist in the field of animal tumors but also a linguist, interpreter at scientific meetings, scientific librarian, cytologist, and authority on chemotherapeutic agents and their effects on tumorous and normal animal tissues. She is especially interested in the relationship of microorganisms to cancerous tissues. Irene has always been a fount of information concerning research in other countries. She kept us abreast of much of the foreign literature. At the Scranton meeting in 1953, her paper entitled, "Studies of Fungoidal Forms Found in Malignancy" discussed fungoidal forms found as contaminants in animal tumors and other types of organisms that seem to have a more specific relationship to cancer. At that time Irene had not worked with the mycobacteriumlike microbe that we were later to designate as *Progenitor Cryptocides*. In later years, after she began to work with the same type of microbes that we were isolating, she did monumental work in fulfilling Koch's postulates with her isolates by increasing production of tumors in mice of known spontaneous tumor incidence.

Irene also demonstrated by her blood-culture method that, of 56 mice that became tumor-bearing during their lifetime, 49, or 93 percent, were carrying the organism in their blood by one year of age. In 1,400 additional mice studied by this method, a very high correlation was established between the presence of the organisms in the blood and the eventual production of tumors.

Irene was often our severest critic, and she maintained and sustained our association with other scientists in the cancer field because of her wide range of acquaintances through her editorship of *Growth* as well as other worldwide contacts. Her work was, in general, confirmatory of ours, and she made many additional contributions.

It was finally the long political arm of Dr. Cornelius P. Rhoads that closed the Newark laboratory. On April 10, 1951, the *Newark Evening News* announced that $750,000 in cancer research funds were given to the Presbyterian Hospital in Newark. The same amount was given to the Memorial Sloan-Kettering Cancer Center in New York, which Dr. Rhoads headed. The trustees of the Black-Stevenson Cancer Foundation had sifted more than five thousand suggestions on how the funds should be distributed. In announcing the grants, the trustees expressed the hope that Presbyterian Hospital in years to come would develop into a leading cancer center. The foundation was set in the estates of two South Orange, N.J., sisters. The accumulated residuary estate of $1,500,000 was left in trust "for the charitable purpose of providing treatment and care both preventive and remedial, for needy persons who may be afflicted or threatened with the disease of cancer." The bequest stemmed from the tragic death from cancer of Mrs. Black's husband, John A. Black, in 1921, only two years after their marriage. It also specified that the funds go to an institution in New Jersey or in New York. There was a five-year deadline for the disbursement of the funds. Another Mr. Black, the brother of the deceased, went to Bill Rose, publisher of the *Newark Evening News*, to make an appeal for help, and the paper then ran the column asking for suggestions.

More than five thousand replies were sent in. The trustees, after much deliberation, decided that the Presbyterian and the Memorial Center hospitals best met the conditions of the estate. In discussing the gift to Presbyterian, the trustees said that "although it is a general hospital as contrasted to the reputation of Memorial Center as the best-known cancer institute in the world, Presbyterian's personnel and associations are adaptable to a degree of specialization in the treatment and prevention of cancer. Presbyterian conducts a cancer clinic and a speech clinic for laryngectomized patients. Cooperative research activities on cancer supported by grants from the Damon Runyon Fund, Abbott Laboratories and the American Cancer Society are being conducted on the premises by the Presbyterian Branch of Rutgers University Bureau of Biological Research." Officials of the two hospitals then gave written agreements pledging faith with the vision of the Black sisters for helping cancer victims. We were not to know how that faith was betrayed for more than a year.

In the meantime we were conducting our animal immunization programs, exhibiting at numerous medical and scientific meetings, and preparing our material for presentation at the Sixth International Congress of Microbiology in Rome. After exhibiting at the American Medical Association Conference in June 1953, we left on August 5 for Europe.

We were received with much cordiality on our arrival in London. In London we presented our papers and discussed them with colleagues who would be participating in the congress. We were particularly interested in meeting with Dr. Emmy Klieneberger-Nobel at the Lister Institute. Dr. Klieneberger-Nobel is the scientist who first described L-forms of bacteria, which are bacterial forms without cell walls. (She called them L-forms for Lister Institute, where she was doing her research.)

While we were in London we spent a day with Dr. Ernest Brieger of the Strangeways Laboratory at Cambridge University. He had worked both in England and in the United States on the filterable forms of the tubercle bacillus by the use of electron microscopy. A number of previous investigators had described a complex life cycle for the tubercle bacillus, among them Leon Grigoraki. However, Grigoraki did not carry the work to the filter-passing stage, nor did he have the electron microscope to demonstrate these forms that are invisible in the light microscope.

We then flew from London to Frankfurt, the nearest air terminal to Bad Kreuznach, where we planned to visit Dr. Wilhelm von Brehmer, who had worked with the same microorganism we called *P. Cryptocides*. (Of course, he called it by another name, *Syphonospora Polymorpha* Von Brehmer.)

The Sixth International Congress of Microbiology took place in Rome from September 6 to 12. Scientists arrived from all over the world, representing many fields of microbiological research. Two Nobel Prize winners, Sir Alexander Fleming and Dr. Selman Waksman, were present, and we eagerly discussed our work with them.

On the afternoon of September 9 our group from the Presbyterian Hospital of Newark, N.J., presented our papers. In summary it can be said that these papers demonstrated the presence of the *P. Cryptocides* in tissues, their cultural properties, their identification as specific microorganisms, and their ability to produce pathogenic lesions in experimental animals. We also demonstrated that immune bodies can be produced that indicate the close relationship of these organisms to one another, whether of human or animal strains, and that the so-called viruses of animal tumors could well be the filterable forms of these causative bacteria. In addition, these microorganisms could produce immune bodies that affect the course of the disease in the infected host.

In the meantime, reports of our papers had been published in several of the newspapers in the United States, such was the prestige of the Rome conference. We were not aware, though, that the *New York Times*, the *Washington Post*, and our own home town newspapers would carry an account of our presentation in Rome. Upon our return, we were met on the dock by several newspaper science reporters who told us that our papers presented in Rome were being challenged.

Here is an example of one report:

NEW YORK DOCTORS CHALLENGE
CANCER GERM REPORT

A spokesman for the New York Academy of Medicine today discounted claims of a medical research team that a cancer-causing microorganism has been isolated and that it has yielded an anticancer serum in animals. The spokesman, Dr. Iago Gladston, executive secretary of the academy's committee on medical information, said the presence of germs in cancerous tissue has been noted before, but these appear to move in after the cancer has developed.

"This is an old story and it has not stood up under investigation," he said. "Microorganisms found in malignant tumors have been found to be secondary invaders and not the primary cause of the malignancy."

The claim was made yesterday in Rome at the Sixth International Congress of Microbiology by a New Jersey research team. They pictured cancer as a generalized disease caused by an organism in the human blood stream, and reported that rabbits and sheep inoculated with an antiserum produced "potent immune bodies." Members of the team were Dr. Virginia Wuerthele-Caspe [now Livingston-Wheeler], *Dr. Eleanor Alexander-Jackson, Dr. L. W. Smith and Dr. G. A. Clark, all associated with Presbyterian Hospital in Newark.*

We had expected a refutation of our work, of course, since in 1953 it was felt that cancer was not an infectious process but a metabolic or deficiency disease. The complex cycle has come full circle again, so that today almost every scientist believes that cancer is an infection but that no specific agent has yet been identified. It was not until our classification at the 1969 New York Academy of Science meetings that we were able to present the full scope of our work to the American scientific world. However, the 1953 newspaper refutations were for the most part inaccurate and merely echoed a lot of the establishment questioning we had been getting all along.

Upon our eventual return to the laboratory, though, we were still exhilarated by our successes in Europe and the recognition we received from world-renowned scientific giants. We were convinced that with our upcoming grant we would finally be able to proceed with the work that would eventually lead to a completely new attitude toward the treatment of cancer; perhaps we would be able to develop our vaccine for its cure.

We were met with the cruel reality of what had transpired behind our backs. As Mr. Hardin, one of the directors of the Black grant, lay dying of cancer in the Memorial Center, he had been prevailed upon to sign a codicil to the bequest stating that we at the Presbyterian Hospital could not expend our share of the grant without the permission of Dr. Rhoads' Memorial Center. As it turned out, the only acquisitions that Dr. Rhoads would grant us were a new wing to be added to the hospital and the installation of *a high-voltage cobalt machine.* The sisters Black were betrayed as were Dr. Alexander-Jackson and myself, who had labored so long and diligently to establish a top-flight research laboratory devoted to the *biological* approach to the treatment of cancer, and *not* to radiation. It was our work that brought the $750,000 gift to Presbyterian in the first place, yet it was the machine this gift purchased that destroyed all that we had accomplished.

At the time of the announcement of the Black grant, we were elated. We could foresee establishing preventive clinics across the nation that would screen patients and immunize them when they were bacteriologically positive, clinics that would promote better life habits, better nutrition, safer and cleaner surroundings, industrial and environmental control of carcinogens, earlier detection of precancerous lesions and genetic counseling.

It was a great dream while it lasted.

7

SAN DIEGO

THE LAST STOP

TEN OF THE MOST productive years of my life had been spent in the Newark area, and it was sad to think it had come to an end. I thought of the babies I had delivered, the many wounds I had sewn up, the patients I had treated and healed, the students and teachers I had met and befriended, the clinics I had attended, the many cancer patients I had cared for . . . and above all, the laboratory in which we had all toiled so tirelessly, with such high hopes and ambitions, now dismantled and never to be opened again. Perhaps when cancer is stamped out for good, just like polio and smallpox, the world will know that much of the pioneering work started in that innovative laboratory in Newark.

I consoled myself with the thought that I was going to join my family in California; my parents and my sister lived there. It was 1953, and we bought a house in Beverly Hills. I became an active member of the Los Angeles County Medical Society, but I couldn't find a research position and had to content myself with work in the L.A. Board of Education's general medical office at Civic Center. The work was interesting, but life on the L.A. freeways was getting me down, so we eventually moved to San Diego where I began work at the San Diego Health Association clinic as a medical internist and clinician. It was at that time that my husband, Dr. Joseph Caspe, died of diabetes and heart disease. I was now almost fifty years old and beginning a totally new life.

The new life was busy indeed. As the only woman at the San Diego clinic and the last physician hired, I worked almost double-time to become accepted by the rest of the staff and to establish my name in the area, as well as to keep my eye open for research opportunities. It was at the clinic that I met Dr. A. M. Livingston, who was head of the Eye, Ear, Nose, Throat and Allergy Department, and, a few years later, in 1957, we were married.

Although I was no longer actively engaged in cancer research, except in the clinical aspect of cancer detection, our papers from the Rome congress had sparked a great deal of interest among other distinguished scientists who believed in the infectious nature of cancer. They also had isolated the pleomorphic microorganism that we called *P. Cryptocides*. Though they were calling it by a number of different names, what they saw was undoubtedly some form of the same causative agent. We had no quarrel with the European investigators. I believed that I was the first investigator to show that the causative organism was an Actinomycetales, which includes the tubercle bacillus, and that the so-called viruses of animal tumors were, in reality, filterable forms of this same organism. Dr. Alexander-Jackson's work in the pleomorphism of the lepra and tubercle bacilli greatly enhanced this concept.

Dr. Alexander-Jackson had become interested in the European group and was appointed the American secretary to the First International Congress for Microbiology of Cancer and Leukemia. A congress was set up in Antwerp, and I was named one of three vice-presidents. Dr. E. Villequez, director of the Central Blood Bank of France and professor of experimental medicine at the University of Dijon, France, was the president. The other vice-presidents were Dr. F. Gerlach, from the University of Vienna, Austria, and Dr. Clara J. Fonti, president of the Centro Internazionale Oncological di Viggio, Milan, Italy.

On Monday, July 14, 1958, the congress convened. The opening began with an address by the president on "Humanism and the Struggle against Cancer." I had the honor of being the first speaker of the scientific session. The papers presented were entirely concerned with the immunological approach to the cancer problem. Again, this material was far in advance of the work being done in the United States. For example, at that time Dr. Robert Huebner of the National Cancer Institute's division of virology had not yet proposed his theory of the C-particle, a noncontagious virus, to be the cause of cancer when activated. This Huebner theory, on which great sums of money would be expended, was very old hat at the very time it was proposed because it had already been presented in Europe. At the afternoon meeting of the congress Dr. Nello Mori, director of the Instituto Microbiologicol Bella Vista, Naples, spoke on "My Conception of the Causative-Pathological Symbiosis of a Certain Parasite in Cancer and Methods of Combating the Parasite by Immunization." Dr. Gerlach spoke on "Latency and Regression of Tumors Brought About by Specific Therapy." Dr. Clara Fonti spoke on the "Pathogenic Etiology of Cancer and Its Treatment." Dr. Eleanor Alexander-Jackson showed her film on the "Morphological Changes in the Human Tubercle Bacillus." Dr. Irene Diller spoke on the "Morphological Changes in Mouse and Rat Blood."

All these distinguished scientists, back in 1958, had been carrying on significant research in the biological and immunological treatment of cancer for years. It is still only now that the United States orthodoxy is beginning to catch up. Because of the suppressive actions of the American Cancer Society, the American Medical Association, and the Food and Drug Administration, our people have not had the advantage of the European research. The deliberate suppression of our work in this country has set cancer research back a number of decades. If the animal immunization studies done by Shope and others in this country had been regarded as prototypes for human immunization, and the early work of Glover, Gregory, and L'Esperance had been taken more seriously, cancer treatment would now be far advanced. This work has been ignored because certain powerful individuals backed by large monetary grants can become the dictators of research and suppress all work that does not promote their interests or that may present a threat to their prestige. Much of this material is documented in *The Cancer Conspiracy* by Robert E. Netterberg and Robert T. Taylor, published by Pinnacle Books in 1981.

Of particular interest to me at the congress was the work of Dr. Fonti. In the autumn of 1958 she wrote a book called *Etiopatogenesi del Cancro*, published by Amedeo Nicola & Co., Milano, which revealed that she had developed a method of staining preserved blood slides so that the presence of the cancer infection could be evaluated in the blood of patients. Her procedures and treatments were thoroughly documented in this book. It is painstakingly written with great accuracy and has many beautiful color illustrations. What impressed me above all was Chapter III on *Autocontagio*, or self-infection. In 1959, Dr. Fonti inoculated the skin on her chest between her breasts with a cancer culture—not with the cells but with the culture. A cancerous growth occurred in the area. This Dr. Fonti removed and had analyzed. The diagnosis revealed that a cancer had been produced through the inoculation of a *bacterial culture*. There is a photograph of the lesion as well as a photomicrograph of the pathological section with the diagnosis of a "basal cell epithelioma." All of us who have studied the microbiology of cancer are convinced that the disease is infectious but not contagious, that is, that it can only be transmitted by direct contact.

Soon after we returned to the United States, our heavy schedule resumed again. Both Dr. Livingston and I worked long hours at the clinic and I suffered a near fatal heart attack and had to curtail my medical activities for a few years while I recuperated.

During this recuperation period Dr. Alexander-Jackson received a grant from the National Institutes of Health (NIH) to continue with the Rous work at the Institute of Comparative Medicine at the College of Physicians and Surgeons of Columbia University. Meanwhile, Dr. Irene Diller and her colleagues at the Institute for Cancer Research in Philadelphia were carrying on corroborative studies of the acid-fast organisms I had first discovered back in 1947. In 1965 Dr. Diller was invited to New Orleans to attend the annual American Cancer Seminar for Science Writers. True to character, Irene gave a fair and impartial presentation of the microbiological approaches to the cancer problem in which we had all collaborated. On March 30, 1965, I was made aware of her report by an article which appeared in the *San Diego Union*. As a result of Irene's presentation, Eleanor and I were invited to present papers at the March 1966 seminar that was held in Phoenix, Arizona. These seminars were initiated as a means of advising the tax-paying, gift-donating public as to what was being done with the money invested in cancer research. The invitation I received was signed by Dr. Harold S. Diehl, senior vice president for research and medical affairs. We also knew that our old friend Patrick McGrady would be in charge of the science writers and their scheduled releases. My husband was generously invited to attend with us. It was considered a great honor to be invited to become a member of the faculty of the seminar, because thereafter the names of the participants were kept permanently on the faculty roster. Mr. McGrady told us that we were scheduled for the last day of the program since our material was quite controversial, and he thought there would be less commotion after our presentations at that time.

This timing of our presentation was undoubtedly wise. Whenever anyone presents a new concept and criticizes the old ones, the proposer must be prepared to stand the "slings and arrows" that invariably follow. I knew what would happen when we stood on the podium and offered our papers. I was placed in the position of proposing new methods of immunological treatment of cancer in humans. I felt like the bull's-eye in the target of a dart game. Before ascending the podium I took the opportunity of slipping away to the ladies' room where I fortified myself with a mild sedative and a heart pill. Then I offered up a silent prayer that there would be ears to hear and minds and hearts that would open to our message.

I had intended only to present the theoretical aspect for determining the cancer-prone individual and to suggest future methods for preventive immunization. Also, I wanted to convince our scientific audience that cancer is an infection, and that surgery, radiation, and chemicals cannot eradicate a continuing infectious process. I stated that a "screening program of the entire population could be undertaken by routine blood cultures to determine the presence of these mycobacteria, correlated with evaluation of blood smears and related to immune competency by various methods of antigen-antibody determination." Both Eleanor and I claimed that this organism had the ability to change its form and might vary its appearance from that of a fungus to that of a cluster of virus-size pleuro-pneumonialike organisms, PPLO, or mycoplasma. I had not intended at that time to discuss some of my earliest efforts in immunizing patients. When I was asked if that were possible, I replied that it was and cited three early cases. Immediately, the press misquoted us and said we had a "cure for cancer" by immunization, even though that was not our main objective in the presentation of our work. In the original presentation I stated that the collagenophilic mycobacteria, which include the cancer organism, have thrown researchers off for years because they are able to change their forms. I also reported that, in a series of breast-cancer studies at the Naval Hospital in San Diego, the best results were obtained with surgery alone, the next best with surgery and radiation, and the worst with surgery, radiation, and chemicals.

I implied that the cobalt machine might reduce the size of the tumors but contributed very little to the long-term cure of the disease. Dr. John Lawrence of the Lawrence Radiation Laboratories (now called the Lawrence Livermore Laboratories) had previously stated that his hope was for a cobalt machine in every town and village in the United States. At that statement I became excited and began to wave a petri dish (used for making cultures) over my head and said that it could be mightier than all the high-powered radiation machines in the world. Nice Dr. Diehl tried to smooth over this statement by saying, "Thousands of patients have been cured by surgery and radiation, but, of course, we hope that research will eventually render these treatments unnecessary."

The Phoenix newspapers were kind. One reported our "basic requirements for formation of the cancer cell to be the causative microorganism and that all other factors such as coal-tar irritants, other microorganisms, the aging process, any chronic irritants leading to poor local resistance and giving rise to immature, susceptible reparative cells, may prepare the soil for the multiplication of the cancer organism and its penetration into the cytoplasm and nucleus of the host." Patrick McGrady said, "It could be they are right. Cynicism has never cured cancer and never will." Dr. Jorgen Fogh, a virologist at the Sloan-Kettering Institute for Cancer Research, said in an interview that he had examined more than 150 cancers, including a dozen leukemias, and had found nothing that resembled mycoplasma or the PPLO.

Meanwhile, Dr. Leon Dmoschowski of the University of Texas Anderson Hospital and Tumor Institute was coming up with evidence that mycoplasma may, indeed, play a part in cancer. It seems that the point of view favored depends on the prestige of the institution rather than on the merits of the research.

Three years later, in the *Journal of the American Medical Association*, July 28, 1969, there was a summary of the work of K. A. Bisset, who wrote in the *New Scientist*, June 12, 1969, that "Various Mycoplasma have been suspected of causing some disease whose etiology is not yet clear." He speculated that many diseases could be caused by mycoplasma or by parts of this elusive bacterium. "The fact that Mycoplasmas can break down into virus-like particles, easily identifiable on electron-microscope examination and similar to those found in the blood of leukemia patients, leads to a strong suspicion that Mycoplasma may be a culprit in the development of certain malignant processes." Also, Dr. Bernard Roswit, reporting in Chicago at the Radiological Society of North America on the year-long study of more than five hundred patients at seventeen Veterans' Administration hospitals, recently stated, "At present it appears that the patient is at the mercy of his cancer and his survival depends more upon the stage of the disease, type of cell and biological character of the cancer than upon the therapeutic act."

The patients in this study were divided into two groups, half receiving the best of radiation treatment and the other half only sugar pills. *At the end of the year only 18 percent of the radiated were alive while 14 percent of those getting sugar pills alone survived.* Those treated lived only thirty days longer than the untreated, and none of the patients in either group was cured. However, Dr. Roswit said the radiation did shrink the tumors temporarily and helped the morale of the patients, but it did not prolong life.

A general uniformity is being forced upon the American public. A doctor who does not conform can lose hospital privileges. If the patient does not conform, insurance carriers may refuse to pay the insurance. Does not each individual have the right to decide what may be done to his or her body? In some hospitals, patients have been put on "double blind studies" where neither they nor their physicians know what treatments they are getting. In certain cases cancer victims have been forced to wear wigs so that no one will know whether a drug is causing their baldness. They are herded like sheep into pens for medical treatment about which they are neither informed nor consulted.

For the three recuperative years following my heart attack in 1962, I was relatively inactive in cancer research but was giving a lot of thought to my future. The seeds of independence were starting to grow once more, and my restlessness added to the beginnings of the idea of opening up my own immunotherapy clinic. I devoted most of my time in that period to teaching mental health and hygiene at Calwestern in Point Loma and to community volunteer work with the San Diego Symphony, the Children's Adoption Society, the Opera Guild, the local Vassar Alumnae Association, the La Jolla Pen Women, and others. During this time something happened which, although I didn't realize it at the time, was probably the event that ultimately resulted in the writing of this book.

A friend who had brought care packages to me when I was in the hospital, Betty O., brought me sad news one day. Her husband, Dr. Ralph O., had a malignant tumor of the thymus gland, which along with the heart and major blood vessels is located in the middle of the chest cavity. His lymphoma was diagnosed as being bigger than a baseball. An operation revealed that there was nothing that could be done, since the tumor had grown into all the surrounding tissues and couldn't be removed. His doctors said that radiation might be temporarily helpful, but were honest in telling him that no one seriously thought he could be helped for long. (I recall making a mental note of a serious car accident he had had a few years earlier that had required large amounts of blood from the local blood bank.)

While telling me about her husband, Betty broke down in tears. Then she looked at me imploringly and blurted, "Oh, Dr. Virginia! You know so much about cancer, and you are always talking so proudly about how you're saving animals from tumors! Can't you do the same thing for my husband? Can't you do *anything* for Ralph?" I was reluctant to undertake treating him, but they were both such dear friends that I agreed to try. Dr. O. became my first human patient.

We treated him with an autogenous vaccine as a nonspecific immune stimulation, mild antibiotics, and diet. He died only recently, of a heart attack, after having lived almost twenty additional years.

Dr. O. was so pleased with his recovery that he put me in touch with a friend of his, a physician in San Diego, with whom I then collaborated on treating the immune systems of a few of his patients, with excellent results. Finally, Dr. O. himself asked one of his patients to give me a grant so that I could continue some of my research. That small grant was then followed by a grant from the Fleet Foundation of San Diego, which continued for several years. Later on, the Fleet grant formed the nucleus of the Livingston Fund at the University of San Diego, which has since moved to the Livingston-Wheeler Medical Clinic. Gifts from patients and friends also kept my research work going.

In order to receive the Fleet grant I had to affiliate with a nonprofit group, so that money could be given tax-free. I chose the San Diego Biomedical Group, an association of scientists consisting of physicians, engineers, and college professors, and I set up a small lab at the Biomedical Institute, where I worked for a year. Simultaneously, I also opened a small office in the neighborhood, which allowed me to consult with a few patients on a research basis. Dr. Eleanor Alexander-Jackson came out to stay with me for a month, and we again went over the work I was doing to reconfirm the presence and cultural properties of the *P. Cryptocides* group. Eventually, when my technician left on maternity leave, I decided I needed larger facilities, so I joined the University of San Diego as associate professor of microbiology.

By the summer of 1968 we had gravitated to what would eventually become the Livingston Medical Clinic. Dr. Alexander-Jackson came out again to stay with us for three months, and in addition to my husband, we had a full-time technician, a medical student, and Dr. Gerhard Wolter from State College working together with us in the USD laboratory. We carried on extensive bacteriological work on *P. Cryptocides*, which led to our landmark group of papers presented at the 1969 meeting of the New York Academy of Sciences, where we formally presented the classification of the cancer-causing microbe.

Dr. Alexander-Jackson acted as chairman for our section, which was called "Microorganisms Associated with Malignancy." For the record, and for readers who may wish to review these papers for technical reasons, I would like to present the authors and titles of our papers. They were: the paper Dr. Alexander-Jackson and I coauthored classifying the microbe; a presentation of a film we had made showing the *P. Cryptocides* organisms living in blood samples of five terminal cancer patients; Dr. Irene Diller's monumental paper "Experiments with Mammalian Tumor Isolates"; and my husband Dr. A. M. Livingston's "Toxic Fractions Obtained from Tumor Isolates and Related Clinical Implications." Dr. Florence Seibert (of tuberculin fame) gave a paper on "Morphological, Biological and Immunological Studies of Isolates from Tumors and Leukemic Bloods," and Dr. Alexander-Jackson then read her Rous paper, "Ultraviolet Spectrogramic Microscope Studies of Rous Sarcoma Virus Cultures in Free Cell Medium."

We were a huge success at the meeting, and our statements about the microbial aspects of cancer were no longer ridiculed. Back at USD we received more than 500 requests from all over the world for reprints of our papers and the articles published in *The Annals of the New York Academy of Sciences*. At least we felt satisfied that our lifetime of knowledge and experience was now on record in the leading science libraries of the world. This is why I just smile when so many cancer physicians today keep asking me, "What scientific papers have you published?" I usually state that I have published more papers than all of them put together, if they would only take the trouble to *look*!

We recently published the *Compendium*, a collection of the above papers, which can be obtained from the Livingston-Wheeler Foundation for the Research of Cancer and Allied Diseases, 3232 Duke Street, San Diego, CA 92110.

Shortly after we returned home from New York, Dr. Livingston and I made the decision to open a clinic that would be available to cancer patients from all over the world. We would treat the immune systems of these patients, bringing all the combined clinical and research experience of decades of work to bear on this horrible disease. The case of Dr. Ralph O., still hale and hearty years after he was declared terminal, encouraged our decision. Today the clinic is still open, providing immunotherapy to hundreds of new patients annually, and having more than an 80 percent rate of success in helping victims of cancer find the path to recovery and a normal, comfortable life span.

8

YOUR
IMMUNE
SYSTEM

YOUR IMMUNE SYSTEM is your defense force, the total protection your body offers against foreign invaders that would contaminate, or infect, your body. The cliché in medicine is to compare the immune system and these "invaders" to military action, with armies, reinforcements and various weaponry. However, it has become a cliché only because it is an accurate analogy and approximates the drama of immune reactions in the body. Your body does, in fact, employ a patrol force, a strike force, a counterattacking army with reinforcements, and even bombs and undercover spies who "mark" the enemy invaders as targets for attack.

The immune system, though complex and designed with redundant backup systems that by comparison would make any sophisticated aerospace computer look as simple as a light switch, is your *only* protection against innumerable afflictions and diseases. It destroys literally thousands of *potentially* disease-causing substances in your body, as well as those substances which we *know* are disease-causing. It also participates in the repair and healing process after an affliction has been eradicated. This heroic immune system protects your body both from within (against the by-products of your biochemical reactions) and without (against pollutants, poisons, etc., from *all* foreign substances and toxic agents, including bacteria, viruses and chemicals). It can discriminate between what is part of your body and what is not; between what is friendly and what is enemy; between what wants to help you and what wants to kill you. If you did not have an immune system, you would die within weeks or else spend your life in a hermetically-sealed plastic oxygen tent.

Perhaps as you are reading this book you have been reminded of the statement currently in vogue: "We all have cancer in our bodies; it's just that our immune system is keeping it in check." If you were to change the statement to: "We all have cancer-causing *bugs* in our bodies," it would be absolutely true. It is our immune system that is keeping us from developing cancer, and it is the breakdown of our immune system that allows cancer to grow.

The quality of your health, both physical and mental, is a good way to measure how strong your immune system is in general. Do you get colds? (Don't say "Everyone does"—many people don't, and it's no accident.) Do you catch every flu bug that comes around? Do you smoke? Do you drink too much? (Don't analyze your social group—everyone knows deep in their heart whether they do or not.) Is your diet one of junk foods, frozen and canned foods, meat and poultry, high in sugar, and devoid of vitamin and mineral supplements? If the answer to these questions is yes, then your immune system is not at its peak strength.

If, on the other hand, you never get sick, if you can visit sick friends and not catch their colds or flus, if you don't smoke, if you drink only moderately, if your diet is high in raw vegetables and low in meat, poultry and junk foods, if you have a substantial vitamin supplement program high in vitamins A, C, and E— then you may be sure your immune system is working at a high strength level.

The reason, then, that you get sick is that your immune system is weak. (As always, remember, there are exceptions—

an especially virulent bug might attack an immunologically strong person and lay the person low, but the immune system is what will fight it off and have the person back on his or her feet quickly, whereas the immunologically weak person will be sick for a long time, perhaps contract other infections or symptoms, and take a long time to recover.)

Cancer is a disease of the immune system. Or, more accurately, it is a disease of a *weak* immune system. Your immunity must drop to a very low level before cancer can grow, and when it drops to an extremely low and weak level the cancer cells start to spread. Your body has no defense against them, or what small defense it has is not enough. The invaders on the beach keep landing more and more troops and marching inland with their machine guns to capture the territory, while your pitifully small and poorly armed resistance force can do nothing to stop the enemy's progress.

Every cancer patient who comes to our clinic has a severely depressed immune system.

It follows, then, that if you maintain a strong and healthy immune system, your chances of ever getting cancer are virtually nil. And the ability of your immune system to successfully prevent cancer is directly dependent on your state of nutrition. If your diet provides all the nutrients needed by your immune system to maintain maximum strength, and if your liver and other organs are producing the proper amounts of enzymes to process these nutrients, the chances are excellent that you will not contract cancer. Little did I expect to find, in my early days of research, that the shortage of a single vitamin or mineral would have drastic effects on immunity. But experiment after experiment, test after test, has shown this to be true. Conversely, *increased* amounts of certain vitamins and minerals can strengthen your resistance to disease.

This is where I get into trouble with the medical profession. There is almost always a knee-jerk reaction against vitamins and minerals—and against the one who is proposing them—on the part of American physicians. Even though the aforementioned study authorized by the National Academy of Sciences concluded that we should eat more foods high in certain vitamins to avoid cancer (they stopped short of recommending supplements), the average doctor still winces when any disease therapy includes a dietary regimen and vitamin supplements. We recommend a lot of vitamin A analogs in the Livingston Anti-Cancer Diet, for both the pre-cancer and post-cancer programs, yet doctors warn their patients that too much vitamin A is toxic. A person taking 10,000 units per day is told to be careful and take only 5,000. A person taking 25,000 units sends the physician into shock. A *cancer* patient, who needs all the vitamin A possible, is given only token amounts of vitamin supplements. But that same physician cannot cite a single instance of vitamin A toxicosis reported in the medical journals and cannot even tell his patient how much is *too* much. The truth is that a healthy adult can take much more than 5,000 units a day without experiencing any toxic effects. The father of my collaborator on this book was dying of cancer of the bladder when his doctor cautioned him against taking too much vitamin C because he "might get kidney stones." The poor man was wasting away and trying to slow down his disease, yet his doctor was worried about an extremely *rare* effect of too much vitamin C! In short, the A.M.A. is still coming out of the Middle Ages on the subject of vitamin supplements. (On the other hand, perhaps if patients and lawyers were not so quick to sue for malpractice, or if there were not so much vitamin quackery, we'd have more enlightened attitudes from our family physicians.)

Most people are now aware that Dr. Linus Pauling, twice Nobel laureate, announced fourteen years ago his thesis that large amounts of ascorbic acid—vitamin C—could prevent and cure the common cold. He contended that vitamin C is an essential ingredient that aids our cells in carrying out a defensive immune process called phagocytosis. (In this process our cells envelop and digest harmful foreign bodies.) Dr. Pauling's experiments showed that higher levels of vitamin C than we normally have in our body tissues could ward off the bugs that give us colds and infections. He was scoffed at by the medical community, and it wasn't until recently that his theory began to be accepted by mainstream doctors.

Before Dr. Pauling's thesis, a biochemist named Dr. Irwin Stone theorized that, by reason of a genetic "accident" millions of years ago, man lost his ability to synthesize a certain enzyme required in the production of ascorbic acid in the body. Hence, man started taking in ascorbic acid exogenously (i.e., from outside sources) by eating leaves, plants, and roots, and today is one of the few mammals on the face of the earth who doesn't manufacture its own ascorbic acid. Therefore, Dr. Stone postulated, we are all walking around with CSS—chronic subclinical scurvy—that is only palliated by our intake of ascorbic acid-bearing foods. (On the other hand, perhaps man started foraging in the forest for plants and leaves and then no longer needed the enzyme to make ascorbic acid, because it was suddenly so plentiful.)

Dr. Pauling, in classic immune system theory, took Dr. Stone's thesis one step further and formulated his vitamin C and the common cold statements. Many scientists have now put forth the proposition that if a little extra vitamin C can boost our immunity and prevent colds and scurvy, then perhaps regular exogenous doses of vitamin C could help our bodies ward off other diseases as well and, in fact, maintain a healthier immune system and a higher level of health in general.

The question now arises: Is being "well" simply not being sick, or are there varying levels of "wellness"? Can we be only a "little bit well" (i.e., just barely not sick), "pretty well," and "very, very well"?

The answer is yes. A person can be only well enough so as not to be sick, or can be extremely well so as to feel absolutely great all the time! And the reason is that the strength or weakness of the immune system determines how you feel—whether you're barely well and will get sick at the drop of a hat, or extremely well and seldom get sick.

IMMUNITY AND
THE DIET CONNECTION

The great changes in American eating patterns over the past several decades are largely responsible for the present high rate of cancer. The modern diet is simply deficient in providing the nutrition essentials that maintain a healthy, vital immunity to cancer. Hence, with these lowered defenses, cancer can start and spread with little or no opposition by our bodies. All too often, what we put into our mouths either causes or directly contributes to the onset of cancer through the depression of our immunity.

It is becoming an old story in these enlightened times, and you've heard it before in books, articles, or TV interviews. We won't belabor it here, but to review it quickly: A century ago, most Americans ate food grown in their own gardens or farms. They picked ripe fruit from the orchard and ate vegetables fresh from the fields. Their food came directly from the garden to their dinner table—and the field itself was chock full of minerals and excellent nutritive soils. Today, most food comes to us from fields hundreds, even thousands, of miles away. Frequently, it reaches our table only after detouring through factories and processing plants, through complex machines that have been devised to peel, cook, and preserve fresh foods, transforming them into bagged, canned, frozen or dried products. Fruits and vegetables are sprayed, waxed, pickled, sweetened, dyed, conditioned and sterilized... and are reduced to only a fraction of the nutrients nature intended by the time we eat them. Every day, Americans consume the contents of more than 90 million cans and jars and more than 40 million pounds of frozen and packaged foods.

The changes in our food, over the past generation alone, are nothing short of frightening.

Let me list just a few:

■ Thirty years ago, the average American ate thirty-one pounds more of fresh fruits and twenty pounds more of fresh vegetables per year.

■ Fifty percent of the processed and packaged foods we eat today didn't exist a decade ago.

■ It is estimated that 80 percent of the packaged food items that will be sold in supermarkets ten years from now do not exist today.

■ As many as 500 new food products are introduced in a given year.

■ The food industry spends approximately $2 billion a year in advertising—mostly to push nutritionally deficient or sugar-laden foods like candy, snacks, soft drinks, fatty foods, and sugared cereals.

An enormous grocery dollar shift has occurred in these past decades toward foods that offer little but calories. People are buying less milk and fewer dairy products and more soft drinks and alcohol. They are consuming less fresh citrus fruit and more frozen juice and lemonade. Instead of eating fresh potatoes, we consume more processed potatoes (frozen, precooked, ready-to-serve items such as potato chips, french fries and instant mashed potatoes). We have been taken in by "convenience foods"—eat-and-run items, filled with starch, sugar, and chemical additives, that offer little or no nutritive value.

While we pride ourselves on being the "best fed" people in history, our diets *rarely* provide us with all the nutrients needed by our bodies and immune systems. It is perhaps the ultimate irony that we are responsible for crippling our own immune systems through nutritional starvation. The "best fed" nation in history also has the highest incidence of cancer and heart disease. What is needed is for everyone to realize that what you eat affects the chances of getting cancer, and that there is a scientifically proven diet that guarantees fortification of the immune system against cancer and other diseases.

YOUR HEALTH
BANK ACCOUNT

Let's look at this a different way. Your immune system is like your "health savings account." Deposits are made in currencies of good food, avoidance of toxic substances, and maintenance of a positive mental outlook. If the immune account has grown as a result of healthy deposits, and the time comes for a "withdrawal," your immune forces can be mobilized to combat disease. However, when your account is overdrawn disease can only gain a foothold. There is no borrowing—your immune system has no credit rating. It is either solvent or broke.

When patients come to our clinic, we test their "immune financial condition" as quickly and accurately as a banker can check a balance in a passbook. Unfortunately, what we find so often in patients with advanced cancer is that their immune systems are bankrupt.

Eating ersatz foods is like depositing play money into your bank account and expecting interest and real money when you make a withdrawal. It simply doesn't work. With the Livingston Anti-Cancer Diet and the discoveries outlined in this book, you will acquire the ability to become an "immunity millionaire."

THE IMMUNE SYSTEM

How your body resists infection, how it rallies the various warrior groups to do battle against the toxic enemies that would like to kill you, is one of the most profound miracles of life. The subject is worth an entire book, and indeed an excellent one has been written for the layperson which explains quite well how your immune system works. I heartily refer you to *The Body Is the Hero*, by Ronald J. Glasser, M.D. (Random House, 1976, 248 pp.). Every cancer patient, and indeed everyone interested in personal health and immunity, should read this outstanding book.

For our purposes here, however, I shall simply try to give an overview of what happens when your body fights infection.

Like the army, navy and air force, there are three important "services" that make up our immune system's defenses: antibodies, granulocytes or white cells, and something with the unusual name of "complement." Let us briefly acquaint ourselves with each system.

The *antibody* system is the army. An antibody is a protein substance in the blood serum that is produced as a reacting agent to attack and destroy an invading foreign body. The foreign substance that incites the antibody's attack is called an *antigen*. This antigen-antibody reaction is generally specific to a certain disease—that is, an antibody will only attack the antigen which instigated its production.

How antibodies work is one of the first miracles of immunity. Each invading body, an attacking microbe, has upon its surface a "marker" which distinguishes it from any other organism, much the same as fingerprints are unique to each individual. These markers are simply molecular configurations of the microbe's membrane. The marker is like the swastika on a WW II German tank or the red ball insignia on the Japanese Zero airplanes. They identified the enemy for our own cannons to shoot at. These markers, which distinguish the antigens, become the identifying insignia for our antibodies to attack. Despite all the dead cells, impurities, broken down bits and pieces of enzymes and hormones, and general microorganic "garbage" continuously flowing through our blood stream, our plasma cells know what's friendly and harmless and what is a "foreign" body bent upon attacking and destroying our tissues.

Newborn babies do not have their own antibodies, and so they use their mothers' to fight early infections. Then, as the baby slowly is exposed to germs that may give it scarlet fever, pneumonia, chicken pox, and typhoid, it creates its own antibodies that attack and neutralize those deadly microbes. When the baby is vaccinated—immunized against specific diseases—it is given an extremely small amount of the antigen disease, thus forming antibodies that attack it and forever keep the immune system fortified against that specific antigen.

The second line of defense in our immunization forces is called *granulocytes*, or granulated white cells. This is our navy. Where the antibodies are our "standing army," ready to be called into action when the invaders launch an attack, the granulocytes are our patrolling P T boats and Coast Guard cutters, constantly mobile, searching the channels of our body for any signs of poisonous material that would do us harm. When this search-and-destroy force does find an invader, it mobilizes millions of troops to attack it relentlessly until it has been destroyed. These white cells are in a constant battle deep inside our blood stream, constantly trying to engulf bacteria and destroy them while the bacteria themselves are constantly emitting their poisons and trying, in turn, to kill our strike forces.

If you were to put a group of granulocytes in a dish of salt water, you would see them casually swimming around, as gracefully as you please, seemingly with no destination and at complete ease. But when you introduce a single bacterium into that tranquil scene, the drama begins as if a starting gun had been sounded. The granulocytes stop, as if alerted by a silent alarm signal to impending danger, and then they begin to prowl through the water, looking for something. Finally they spot it and unleash their terror upon the bacterium with a ferocity unmatched in the animal world. They swarm against the invader, grabbing it and emptying their granules into the cell until it is killed, as if pumping thousands of shells into a single enemy ship.

But the granulocyte strike force only carries light armament. When they come upon an especially tough invader, one with its own army of millions of bacteria, they empty their ammunition into as many invaders as possible, but at the same time know enough to call for reinforcements: the battleships and aircraft carriers of the macrophages.

A *macrophage* is simply a larger, stronger white blood cell. Together with the granulocytes these stronger forces enter the battle and attack relentlessly, to the death. There is no surrender, no negotiation, no standoff. One force wins, and only when its opposition is *totally* destroyed, when not one single cell exists to raise even the weakest resistance. If the invading disease has been reduced from millions of bacteria to a single cell, the armada of granulocytes and macrophages fights on, until that last solitary bacterium has been destroyed. Indeed, even if the enemy wins— as in the case of the person dying of cancer—even if there were only a single macrophage left in the body, it would throw itself into the battle against the overwhelming forces of death, as if it were the last remaining suicide warrior. These white cells are the most loyal and dedicated warriors of all.

The third part of our immune defense is our air force bombers, our armor-piercing shells that actually blow up an invader, as if throwing a hand grenade into the enemy cell. These are called *complement*, a group of nine proteins in our serum that are actually manufactured by the liver (yet another amazingly critical function of this incredible organ). The unique thing with complement is that it is so fierce in its intent to blow up *something* that it cannot differentiate between friend or foe. It will bomb anything in sight, healthy cells as well as invading, poisonous ones. Consequently, it needs a "bombsight," a scout to tell it whom to attack and whom to leave alone.

This brings us back to the antibodies. The antibody is like an advance foot soldier who, while shooting at the enemy, is also signaling messages to air support, detailing exactly where to drop their bombs. As the antibody attaches to the marker on the antigen, it also activates the nearest passing unit of complement, which is the first of the nine component proteins. The complement then attaches to the antibody, which in turn signals the second unit of complement to attach to the cell wall. This continues until the ninth unit of complement attaches to the cell wall, at which time the invading cell is blown to smithereens.

To conclude our simplified comparison of the immune system with military action, these three defensive "services," the army, navy and air force of our immunity, are, of course, run by the Pentagon. Every action is analyzed, and orders are sent to mobilize our various battle forces by the lymph system, the Pentagon of our bodies.

The lymph nodes located throughout our bodies (near our organs, armpits, knees, skin, and practically everywhere) secrete lymphocytes, cells which travel around the body and then return to the lymph nodes. This cycle is continuous. A lymphocyte has no particular locomotive mechanism of its own, yet it lets itself get carried along in the blood stream, through tissues and organs, muscles and skin, until it eventually gets back to the nearest lymph node, passes through it, and then goes out upon its travels once again. This goes on and on, with some form of the lymphocytes, unlike the granulocytes and macrophages, continuing to live for months and years, making their inspection patrols hundreds of times a day. They apparently do not die, and it is thought by some scientists that they may even live as long as we do. The science of immunology is so young that we still don't understand exactly *why* a lot of the actions of our immune systems happen. But the lymphocytes make their inevitable rounds day by day, seemingly innocuous, not doing anything but floating through our bodies, bumping along in the traffic of billions of blood cells.

However, our entire immunology is controlled by these lymphocytes. When a bacterium enters your body, say through a cut on your finger or stepping on a nail at the beach, the antibodies already existing in your system will attack it and prevent infection. Or, if an infection has gained a foothold the entire system of armed forces will attack and fight it, with the dead bodies forming pus at the site of the battle.

When a new invader appears, one that hasn't been in the body before, it will eventually brush up against one of these circulating lymphocytes. And when it does, that lymphocyte gets excited—so excited that during its brief contact with the invader it makes a "print" or a copy of that antigen's marker and rushes to the nearest lymph node with the information. It is as if a messenger has discovered a spy in the midst of our troops, taken a picture, and rushed to the general to announce the news. The general in the war room, the lymph node, then alerts the entire system. He mobilizes the antibodies and flashes the picture of the marker to them; he alerts the P T-boat navy of granulocytes and their backup battleships, the macrophages, and sends them toward the battle site; he makes sure our bombers, the complement, are getting the proper identification information from the antibodies when they make contact with the antigen. And against especially tough enemies, viruses and parasites that may have strong protective shells around them because they are intracellular microbes (such as the *Progenitor Cryptocides* microbe), we even have Green Berets—specially trained "killer" lymphocytes that can attack the invader all by themselves!

As I said, this is an extremely simplified explanation of what is going on within our immune systems, and indeed it can be fun for the sake of instruction to relate it all to a military battle. The main message is that in the final analysis *you* determine whether your forces are well equipped to fight. It is your nutrition that manufactures the ammunition necessary for the weapons to work properly. And it is the vaccine that we administer at our clinic in San Diego that shouts, *"Cancer! Cancer!"* to the generals in the war room.

9

CHICKEN: CANCER IN EVERY POT

AFTER YEARS OF research, I consider the potential for cancer in chickens to be almost one hundred percent. That is, most of the chickens on the dining tables and barbecue grills of America today have the pathogenic form of the PC microbe, which I contend is transmissible to human beings. This is not to be confused with the *dormant* form of the PC in the healthy, high-immunity human being; the PC viral forms in chickens are already pathogenic, generating malignant cells and already forming tumors. Not only that, but many of the chickens processed for human consumption have *already* displayed tumors both visible and invisible to the naked eye but because of hurried processing techniques have sped by inspectors on the production lines.

It has been estimated by Elizabeth Alleen McCulloch, an animal husbandry expert who has been following the incidence of Marek's Disease and other forms of avian leukosis for more than thirty years, that forty percent of human cancers are caused by this pervasive cancer in the chicken population.

And I agree with her, for even though the PC microbe in the healthy human being goes dormant and does not secrete uncontrolled CG after birth, repeated ingestion of the pathogenic PC form in infected chickens and eggs can very well initiate carcinogenic activity in low-immunity persons and begin to form malignant cells.

In 1972, television viewers in Southern California were treated to the news of the burning of thousands upon thousands of chickens because of a local epidemic of Newcastle disease in poultry. (Newcastle disease is a virus affecting the respiratory and nervous systems of birds.) The outbreak was serious enough to be compared with the outbreak of a new strain of influenza among human beings, as far as effective vaccination was concerned. Authorities worked long and hard to eliminate the Newcastle infections, and consumers were leaving eggs and chickens on supermarket shelves in fear of contamination. Prices plunged.

However, the Newcastle disease, although killing thousands of chickens, wasn't nearly the threat to human life as was—and still is—the alarmingly high incidence of cancer in poultry. On February 10, 1970, the *Wall Street Journal* headlined a report: "Chicken Cancer Called Widespread Enough to Pose 'Nightmares' for Poultry Industry." Then in 1971 a controversy erupted about how safe it was to eat chickens. A Department of Agriculture advisory panel had reported that the government ought to relax standards for inspection of poultry affected by leukosis-complex (cancer) diseases. It was contended, at the time, that there wasn't any known connection between the leukosis viruses and human health.

Now, in 1983, we know that this simply is not true. We have shown over and over again in our San Diego laboratories that there definitely is a strong connection between chicken cancers and cancers in human beings. Dr. Peyton Rous, whom we have mentioned often as the Nobel laureate and father of the theory of infectivity of chicken cancer, demonstrated years ago that a certain infectious material he called a "tumor agent" definitely was transmissible.

This was published as far back as 1910 in the *Journal of Experimental Medicine* and in 1911 in the *Journal of the American Medical Association*. Dr. Rous, who spent his career in the laboratories of the Rockefeller Institute for Medical Research, New York, prior to winning his Nobel Prize, contended that ninety-five percent of the chickens for sale in New York City were cancerous. He continued to confirm and reconfirm his findings on the transmissability of chicken cancer for more than fifty years, and made it the subject of his Nobel Lecture on December 13, 1966.

In the *International Review of Experimental Pathology*, 16; 59-154, 1976, Payne, Frazier and Powell discuss the transmissability of a form of chicken cancer called Marek's Disease. They state that annual losses by the poultry industry in the late 1960s was 200 million dollars and that "1.5 percent of broiler carcasses were condemned because of leukotic tumors. In laying and breeding flocks, 10-15 percent mortality was common, and losses up to 80 percent of the flock could be encountered. These heavy losses were the consequence of the acute pathogenic form of Marek's Disease..."

These incidences of chickens condemned because of tumors—up to 60 percent—represent only the tumors that were *visible*. This is one reason why I contend that almost all chickens and eggs available for consumption today have the pathogenic form of the PC, visible or not.

The Rous agent is not a true virus, which needs living cells to survive. Instead, the "tumor agent" could be dried and stored at room temperature for months and even years, and later be placed in solution and injected into susceptible chickens, *who then all developed cancer*.

In my early days of research at the Presbyterian Hospital under the auspices of Rutgers University, I theorized that the Rous tumor was the prototype of all other tumors in humans and animals. Our research group spent several years growing the "tumor agent" in synthetic culture media and through various complex medical-mechanical procedures became satisfied that it was not a virus. We even filtered the cultures, not the extracts of the tumors, through bacteria-restraining filters and studied these under the electron microscope with Dr. Hillier at Princeton. They were *definitely* not viruses.

In our work at Rutgers with the "tumor agent," we kept the cultures, in which there was no visible form of life, incubated them at 37° C, and from these seemingly clear broths there arose the bacterial and fungal stages of the *Progenitor Cryptocides* microbe. We performed this experiment not once but dozens of times, until Dr. James Hillier, with his electron microscope, was satisfied that we had ruled out any contamination that might account for the bacterial growth on incubation. It was a tedious but exciting process in which we learned that a so-called virus could, and did, "convert" to bacterium that had not only submicroscopic forms but also bacillary and coccal (round) forms, and that the bacterium could also develop funguslike stages and spores. On studying the growth of the tubercle bacillus, these stages were entirely comparable to the *P. Cryptocides*.

However, if the Rous agent is not a virus, then there should be both RNA and DNA in the tumor agent as there are in bacterial growths. (Viruses are classified as *either* RNA or DNA; bacteria contain both.) Eleanor Alexander-Jackson's paper "Ultraviolet Spectrogramic Microscope Studies of Rous Sarcoma Virus Cultured in Cell-free Medium" demonstrates that there *is* DNA present in the Rous tumor agent. Since DNA is the master molecule of heredity, it has been easy for virologists to speculate on how a DNA virus could transform normal cells to cancerous ones, but they could not understand how an RNA virus could do this. It seems now that RNA can direct the formation of DNA and probably vice versa. (This was later proven by H. M. Temin, who found an enzyme that transcribes the RNA virus message into DNA. It is called polymerase transcriptase.)

When we compared the cultures obtained from human cancers with those from chicken tumors, there was no discernible difference: the growth pattern of the chicken cancer isolates and that of human cancers were the same. They grew in the same kind of broth in the same way, and they appeared the same in chicken and human tissues. They had the same staining properties with the Ziehl-Neelsen dye. We then did the sheep immunization studies in which we found significant cross-agglutination between the Rous sarcoma, fowl leukosis, and various strains of human cancers. When we injected the isolated cultures into mice, the same kind of diseased lesions developed. In every way, the Rous agent appeared to be a prototype for human cancer. The next step was the immunization of rabbits with the leukosis agent and the use of the antiserum to cure chickens dying of fowl leukosis.

Dr. Bruce W. Calnek, a veterinary researcher at Cornell University, says, "We have no evidence of danger to humans and think there is none whatsoever." However, Dr. J. Spencer Munroe, a New York University professor, injected a laboratory-developed leukosis virus into monkeys in 1963 and found the monkeys developed tumors. He feels the subject needs more research.

Several years ago, a turkey herpes-type "virus" was developed for the control of Marek's disease (a cancerous poultry disease); it is a live microorganism. Its proponents claim that the poultry are protected against Marek's disease, and that the appearance and numbers of tumors are diminished. However, it does not appear to affect the Rous type of cancers and some of the tumors of the older birds. In addition, the leukosis microbe may only be masked by the turkey herpes-type "virus," so that while the tumor response is suppressed the chickens are harboring not only chicken leukosis but also the turkey herpes-type "virus" in addition to whatever other cancer "viruses" they may have. Regardless, there is no doubt that the Rous sarcoma virus is transmissible to the ape. What is man but a fellow primate?

Some have argued that the hydrochloric acid of the human stomach will destroy these cancer agents, especially when they are also acted upon by the enzymes of the digestive tract. However, as the acidity of the stomach decreases with aging, more and more microorganisms are found in the gastric contents from the age of forty upward. The intestinal tract consists of a large bed of absorbing glands and blood vessels, and there is no reason to suppose that the intestinal mucosa differentially rejects the tumor agents and their toxic products. Quite the contrary is true. In our experimental animals that were sacrificed after being infected orally by the tumor cultures, the specific tumor agents were found not only in the living cells of the intestine but also in the small blood vessels and connective tissue layers. It is well known that the Bittner mammary factor in the mouse is transmitted through the mother mouse's milk. There are many diseases that are contracted through ingestion, such as the *Salmonella* group, which contains the typhoid organisms. Incidentally, the salmonella are also carried in the chicken's egg. On occasion, friends have brought me eggs that looked "not right." Often I was able to recover cultures of the *Cryptocides* from them. As one veterinarian said in an interview, "Whatever the hen has is transmitted to the egg as through a sieve."

The question is often asked, "Doesn't cooking destroy the microbes?" I am certain that cooking does destroy many of them. The bacterial stage of the organism dies at 140°F after fifteen minutes. But when a chicken is broiled it is questionable if that degree of heat is attained around the bones. (Many Japanese and Chinese dishes are prepared by cooking the chicken for only five or six minutes.) Another consideration is that during preparation chickens are often washed in the sink where dishes are washed, or placed on kitchen counters where bread is cut or other raw foods are served, and microorganisms can infect these other foodstuffs. I think we have to say that the microbes are not killed by *ordinary* cooking. And some forms of the microbe require sterilization on three successive days of autoclaving for twenty minutes under steam pressure of thirty pounds in order to kill them.

There is no knowledge as yet as to whether cooking detoxifies the microbes that are present in the infected bird. And don't forget that, since the cancer organisms are transmitted to the egg, the usual cooking temperature of soft boiled or scrambled eggs probably does not destroy them. If you must eat eggs, I recommend only well-cooked fried eggs or hard boiled eggs. But even then, I believe there is some risk. The organisms can multiply even under ordinary refrigeration, so stored poultry and eggs may incubate increasing numbers of the agents.

"This is a very, very serious problem," says Ralph Nader, the consumer crusader. He acknowledges that the evidence for transmissibility of fowl disease to man needs much more research but, he says, "There also isn't any proof to show the disease can't be transmitted. And the research on this has been very recent and not thorough at all." He also said that there are insufficient numbers of inspectors, so that "a lot of bad poultry is probably slipping onto your dinner table."

An article a few years ago in the *San Diego Union* was entitled, "Leukosis in Every Pot."

The U.S. Department of Agriculture may be on sound medical ground when it contemplates permitted sale of poultry displaying the evidence of chicken cancer because no definite proof of a link between chicken cancer and human cancer has been proven.

Nevertheless it does not help much for the department to assure us that should the tumor be on a drumstick the diseased leg would be ground up for frankfurters. Somehow, it is not even comforting to learn that most poultry, including that we have been eating, is infected with leukosis to some degree. Considering the furor over cyclamates and the Pill, the proposal to relax the existing ban is, to put it mildly, incredible—and inedible.

There *are* some small tumor-free poultry flocks in our country, but they are rare. Recently the Livingston-Wheeler Medical Clinic obtained a patent on a new chicken/fowl vaccine, and we are now licensed to test it on chickens in California.

Perhaps the government should put off another space shuttle voyage and clean up the poultry industry, whatever the cost.

10
THE LIVINGSTON-WHEELER MEDICAL CLINIC

EVERY YEAR WE TREAT hundreds of patients at our clinic in San Diego. I really do not have an accurate count of *precisely* how many patients we have treated since opening our doors in 1969, but it is well over ten thousand. Our unusually high success rate is based on what I referred to in Chapter Two as our "usual therapy" or our "standard program." This chapter will summarize exactly what happens when a patient comes through our doors.

Our clinic is an outpatient facility. This means that we do not have overnight beds for patients; hence they must make arrangements at local motels, hotels, trailer courts, etc., preferably with kitchen facilities. (We are currently trying to raise funds to purchase an "in care" facility where patients may be supervised, housed, provided with prescribed food, and generally instructed in a warm, friendly atmosphere.)

Since almost all of our patients first make contact with the clinic by telephone, we usually mail them an information pamphlet in order to familiarize them with the clinic and the local environs. The information pamphlet includes biographical information about Dr. Wheeler and me; a summary of our immunotherapy protocol, including a synopsis of our treatment program of vaccines, diet, and vitamins and minerals; a request that the patient secure personal medical records and bring them, or else have pertinent records, such as X rays, mailed to us by the patient's attending physician; a suggestion that the patient bring a companion, in order that the companion may also be instructed by our nurses on the use of medications, injections, and the proper preparation of special foods; an explanation of what an autogenous vaccine is; a checklist of exactly what to expect in the way of conferences with other physicians, diagnostic measures, and conventional treatments; a suggested reading list; a map of the area and a list of accommodations and rates available; and an explanation of financial arrangements so that the patients will know how to check up on their insurance coverage, etc.

After arriving at the clinic, the patient knows immediately that here is a place where *everyone* involved cares about the patient's well-being and comfort. Whenever a patient comes to a physician for advice and help, the physicians are obligated to give unreservedly to that patient the total benefit of their knowledge and skill. Patients often come to us in desperation, knowing that their lives are threatened by a killer disease that has been popularized as having no known cure. The physician must then receive those patients with love and devotion as well as scientific experience. The patient must feel that respect and concern are just as much a part of the treatment as any medication or examination.

A new patient is initially interviewed by either Dr. Owen Wheeler or one of our other highly trained physicians. This meeting is quite extensive, because we try not only to get a comprehensive personal history but also to familiarize the patient further with what can be expected from the immunotherapy program. We even tell the patient what kind of success we have had with any particular kind of cancer. We try to establish an orderly, analytical, and objective but sympathetic, communication line with the patient as we are learning as much as possible.

Everyone who has gone to a doctor knows about giving a history, and we encourage the new patient to write out as complete a historical record as possible before the interview starts. Family background is important, because diseases such as diabetes and cancer are considered to be hereditary. Many other points of a nonmedical nature are also important: Did the patient have a happy home life as a child? A good marriage? Favorite foods? Religious attitudes? Occupation? Cheerful or dour? Will to live or death wish? This is all discussed at the initial interview.

The patient is then examined physically. Careful notes are taken concerning the course of the disease. All conventional methods of diagnosis are employed, including blood counts, urinalysis, blood chemistry, determination of electrolytic balance, kinds, types, and amounts of circulating antibodies, thyroid function, blood proteins, steroid levels, and various tests for collagen diseases. Radioisotope scans of liver, brain, or thyroid are ordered if indicated, as well as mammography, photography, or thermography for breast pathology; multiple transverse echograms for delineating the presence of masses in the abdomen; contrast dye studies for gallbladder, lymphatics, or kidneys; and diagnostic X rays as needed. All these modalities are employed in order to evaluate the patient's disease and to help ascertain what method of treatment will be most efficacious. For special procedures and tests the patient is referred to the many excellent specialists we are fortunate to have in the San Diego area.

The patient is also invited to view videotapes we have prepared on the story of the research work and operation of the clinic. Additionally, the patient begins instruction in our kitchen laboratory in preparing certain foods and operating a juicer.

Meals are provided often in the lounge.

Although immunotherapy is the hope of the future for supplanting the present-day methods of treatment such as surgery, radiation, and chemical blockers of cell replication, the proven methods must be given the opportunity to make their contribution. Established diagnostic techniques must be employed because they represent the accumulation of knowledge up to the present time. Perhaps some day soon there will be a simple serological test for the detection of cancer, such as the Wassermann test for syphilis. Perhaps a single cure will be found, such as penicillin for syphilis. Perhaps an antibiotic will be developed to work against the *P. Cryptocides* microbe. Unfortunately, that time has not yet arrived. However, the main failures of conventional cancer treatment have spurred the entire scientific world to a search for better methods.

When the patient comes to our clinic, we employ the following procedures:

1. A clean-catch urine specimen is obtained from the patient on arrival. This urine is cultured, and the *P. Cryptocides* organisms are isolated and used to prepare an autogenous vaccine. This takes about three weeks. The numbers and kinds of this specific bacterial agent are very important, whether hemolytic or confluent, increasing or decreasing in numbers after treatment.
2. The microbial isolates are also used to perform an antibiotic sensitivity test to determine which antibiotics might help the patient.
3. A urine culture is made twice a week in the beginning in order to determine the numbers and characteristics of the colonies, and whether the antibiotics that have been selected are still effective, or whether they have developed bacterial resistance, in which case a new antibiotic must be chosen.
4. Dark-field and bright-field microscope examinations with supravital staining of a fresh blood droplet are done on every visit. Here again is where the *P. Cryptocides* microbe is seen circulating in the patient's blood, a simple test that is performed routinely for monitoring the progress of the treatment. The dark-field microscope, admittedly, is thought of mostly as a research tool and is more expensive than the conventional bright-field microscope most of us have looked into at one time or another. However, in Europe it is a common instrument in the office of every doctor who pur-

ports to study or treat cancer, and blood is not transfused without first examining it under a dark-field microscope. (During a debate, I recently asked a prominent Los Angeles oncologist when was the last time he looked into a dark-field microscope, and he answered, "In medical school.")

The advanced cancer patient has many pleomorphic forms of the *P. Cryptocides* in his or her blood in vast numbers due to the loss of immunity. Only time and experience can teach an investigator how to read these slides, but almost anyone with some bacteriological experience can learn this procedure with practice. Von Brehmer, Fonti, Villequez, Mori, Freiberg, and Enderlein all employed the examination of fresh blood by dark-field as a method of following the patient's stage of immunity and the course of the disease. With our present knowledge of motile rods, L-forms, mesosomes, spheroplasts, protoplasts, and tubular bodies and spicules these evolutionary forms of the *P. Cryptocides* are better understood.

TREATMENT

1. All poultry products are eliminated from the diet, including eggs as used in baking, because some microbial bodies as well as toxic fractions may survive heating. All sugars are also eliminated, since the *P. Cryptocides* microbes multiply in great numbers during fermentation of sugars and starches, such as those present in candy, cake, ice cream, pastries, and carbonated drinks, all of which may "feed the bugs." Microbes *love* sugar, iron, and copper. (Iron deficiency in a cancer patient is a defense mechanism and a sign that something else is wrong, not a disease in itself.) Overpurified foods such as white flour are also forbidden, since recent research has shown them to be lacking in good nutritive elements. Processed foods, such as those that are

canned, smoked or salted, are eliminated. Raw, fresh, un-adulterated, natural foods are emphasized.

2. Smoking is stopped because tobacco is a known carcinogen. Alcohol is also not allowed, because the detoxification of alcohol puts a tremendous strain upon the liver, which must be restored to peak performance in order to produce the enzymes for vitamin A metabolism as well as essential proteins and to act as a storage center for energy products.

3. A suitable diet is prescribed. (This along with menu plans and recipes will be covered in the next chapter.)

4. We recommend fresh whole-blood transfusion from a young, healthy individual, preferably a member of the family when possible. No blood-bank blood is used unless absolutely necessary. Stored blood loses much of its efficacy in many functions, such as oxygen-carrying power, enzyme activity, antibodies, and effective white blood cells. Also, if there are infectious agents in the blood, such as *P. Cryptocides*, these may multiply during storage. If the patient is not too acutely ill, transfusion may not be necessary. Often sufficient amounts of good fresh blood will cause a tremendous upswing in the sense of well-being due to the rise in oxygenation and fresh antibodies.

5. We use gamma globulin, often of placental origin, as a source of antibodies. Where transfusions are not given, gamma globulin can be given in large doses, as in the cases of the leukemic, sarcoid, or lymphomatous patient. If a loading dose is not given to maximize the patient's antibodies quickly, then 3 cc can be given one to three times a week.

6. Splenic extract is given in 2–5 cc doses two or three times a week. This material is nonallergenic and serves to increase the white blood count. Also, spleen is known to enhance immunogenic systems. Fresh spleen has been observed to cause remission in some cancerous patients. The intact spleen acts to cleanse the blood by removing the intracell-ular parasites that circulate in the red cells. In Hodgkin's

disease the spleen often becomes secondarily infected and is surgically removed for the same reasons that chronically diseased tonsils are removed. However, splenectomy should be avoided whenever possible, especially the removal of a healthy spleen for staging (classifying) Hodgkin's disease.

7. A BCG vaccine is used to stimulate the patient's immune system immediately against the *P. Cryptocides* microbe. BCG, which stands for Bacillus Calmette-Guérin, is an attentuated bovine tubercle bacillus, a close relative of the *P. Cryptocides*. A tuberculin test is administered to see whether the patient has immunity to the tubercle bacillus or has been previously infected with TB. Often patients will state that they have been positive in the past. A recent test showing them to be negative indicates a change in their immune state. If they are negative, BCG can be given in a single dose intracutaneously by the multiple tine method. The reaction is carefully watched as it may serve as a guide for further treatment with vaccines of various kinds. Sometimes a markedly positive vaccination may cause the flare-up of a small tumor and cause it to swell or discharge. The patient is retested in three months by purified protein derivative (PPD). The PPD, if positive, may indicate active tuberculosis, in which case BCG is not given. TB and cancer are seldom seen together. BCG produces mild TB, protective against cancer. If the patient's reaction is only mild, the BCG may be repeated if the original site has faded.

In Chicago, when 85,000 babies were vaccinated against TB and compared over the course of 20 years with babies who were not vaccinated, the vaccinated babies represented only one-tenth of the total deaths from leukemia. BCG also triggers remissions in melanoma, an almost universally fatal cancer of the skin and internal organs. It raises immunity in general against cancer when used carefully in well-controlled doses.

8. Small increasing dosages of nonspecific vaccines may be used. These can consist of bacteria from teeth or tonsils, or can be common respiratory bacteria. These are also useful in treating arthritis. They all serve to control chronic recurrent infections such as colds, which lower resistance.

9. Vitamin B-6, B-12, liver, and multiple vitamins are given and we administer intravenous vitamin C when appropriate. We believe that vitamins A, C and E are effective anticancer nutrients.

10. When the autogenous vaccine is ready it is administered subcutaneously and orally. Reactions must be watched for very carefully so that the patient is not overdosed. Overdosing might, though rarely, result in a mild fever or aching of joints and muscles.

11. The antibiotic program is extremely important. If the right antibiotic is selected and administered in standard doses, the tumors themselves can diminish in size. Some investigators claim this effect is due to concomitant nonspecific infection of the tumor mass, which responds to the antibiotic. However, generally, antibiotics decrease the number of *P. Cryptocides* circulating in the blood. We do not use toxic antibiotics. Frequently, we use bicillin, penicillin G, or ampicillin in large doses for long periods. One patient in a remission from inoperable sarcoma of the neck was on erythromycin for four and a half years. His disease is entirely under control, and he works daily as a longshoreman. Ampicillin administered orally is very useful, and lincomycin and cephgalothin are useful on a short-term basis. Mandelamine is a good medication to give with the other antibiotics. The furadantins can also be helpful. Each case must be carefully evaluated by blood examination and urine culture, followed by frequent sensitivity tests. It must be borne in mind that the kidneys act as a sieve, not only in excreting metabolic waste products but in filtering out bacteria that have entered the blood stream from tumors or

established colonies in the intestinal tract or prostate. Sometimes the urinary tract excretes many of these organisms due to direct infection; this can be determined by culture.

12. We acidify the blood and urine, since a state of imbalance toward the alkaline side is known to exist in tumor patients. Hydrochloric acid in various forms can be given. The acidity of the urine is checked frequently with Nitrazine paper because the healthy stomach secretes large amounts of hydrochloric acid (HCL) during digestion, whereas frequently the cancer patient cannot produce the essential HCL for protein digestion. The patient is advised to keep the urine in the acid range of a pH of 6 or below. (You can buy Nitrazine paper in a drugstore and periodically check your own urine. If the paper turns blue and is alkaline, it means your stomach does not contain sufficient hydrochloric acid, which can mean that your gastric mucosa isn't functioning well, which ultimately can mean that the digestive process is sequentially impaired.)

We also prescribe trace minerals, especially organic iodine (such as is contained in kelp), since iodine is essential in the metabolism of thyroid, the oxidative hormone. Additional thyroid is also given whenever tolerated. The suppressive hormones are prescribed in courses where they have been shown to be helpful, such as stilbestrol in male prostatic disease, and nonmasculinizing synthetic androgen, such as tamoxifen, in women with hormone dependent tumors. However, their use is often self-limited as to long-continuing efficacy. Steroids are used very cautiously to suppress the swelling of tumors during therapy, especially in brain tumors. Probably dexamethasone is the least inhibitory in its action on immunity. Many other supportive measures are given as indicated, such as fresh blood transfusions, tumor necrosing factor, blood washing, and the use of various fractions, such as lysozyme, interferon, complement, Burton blood fractions, hybridomas, and antisera to tumors.

A major discovery I made in 1974 has a great bearing on our treatment program and has already markedly influenced the basic research in cancer throughout the world. This discovery was that the microbe *P. Cryptocides* secretes a mammalian hormone called choriogonadotropin (CG). This is important because CG is a hormone necessary for life itself to begin. It has been shown by Hernan Acevedo, Ph.D., that all cancer cells contain CG, regardless of whether they are animal or human. The CG in the cancer cell is located in the nuclear membrane, the cytoplasm, and the cell membrane. It is postulated that the *P. Cryptocides* may have hybridized with the mammalian nucleus and imparted to the latter the ability to produce CG. In other words the DNA of the *P. Cryptocides* may act as a kind of fertilization of the human or animal cell to initiate an abnormal cell replication, known as cancer.

There are four sources of CG in the human being: the sperm, the trophoblast, the bone marrow, and the cancer cell (via the *P. Cryptocides* microbe). Unless CG is controlled by antibodies, white cells, and dietary factors, it can continue its reproductive activity indefinitely in an uncontrolled way. The reparative cell is also controlled by CG. *All reproductive life, whether of the fetus in utero or of the cancer cell, is controlled by CG.* It is, therefore, the hormone of life and the hormone of death.

That is when the sperm enters the ovum, the secretion of CG by the *P. Cryptocides* microbe envelops the new life cell (zygote) so that the mother's immune system does not reject the fetus. The placenta is coated with CG, protecting the fetus from the mother's immune system and the mother from invasion by the fetal cells. Therefore, when one considers that the *P. Cryptocides* microbe is carried by human sperm and is required for every new life to evolve and survive (because it is the source of the CG), it is not difficult to understand how this potentially killing but also reparative microbe exists in all human cells. However, the microbe remains dormant until our immune systems become so weak as to let it gain a foothold, at which time its secretion of CG allows a tumor to grow. Every tumor has large amounts of CG because of uncontrolled proliferation.

I discovered that abscisic acid, a plant hormone also called *dormin*, a retinoid, or vitamin A analog, plays a regulatory role in the production of CG by the *P. Cryptocides* microbe. This may be the reason that foods rich in the vitamin A analogs, the retinoids and abscisins, appear to have a beneficial action in controlling cancer susceptibility and may even have a regulatory action. Combined with immunization using the whole *P. Cryptocides* vaccine or fractions thereof, such as trehalase or cord factor, there is marked inhibition of the development of tumors in mice.

The practice of surgical oophorectomy, adrenalectomy, hypophysectomy and orchiectomy can only be decried. These are temporary measures and can have no lasting benefit. The reason · there is temporary alleviation is that the end organs such as the ovary, adrenal, hypophysis, and testes are receptors of CG produced by the *P. Cryptocides*. Permanent results obtained by direct attack on the *P. Cryptocides* and on CG, as well as the use of neutralizing factors such as antibodies, immunization, and abscisic acid, have the potential of producing long-term remission or cure without the above surgeries.

We feel that any positive approach that builds the patient's morale is valuable, but we do not advocate any particular method. By paying strict attention to all the details of the treatment, much can be done to alleviate the disease and in many cases point the way to resumption of a useful, active, and happy life.

11
THE ANTI-CANCER DIET

LIVING FOOD, meaning non-processed, fresh vegetables and fruits, with their seeds and nuts, contains all the essentials for good health and good immunity. It is one of the most overlooked preventive medicine resources we have. When food is processed, altered, or adulterated, the health and life-giving factors are markedly diminished. Processed foods provide calories, but they cannot sustain other needs that can only be met by living food. *One of the most vital systems of the body that cannot be sustained by devitalized, dead food is the immune system.*

Today, more than ever before, physicians and scientists worldwide are realizing that the unwholesomeness of our modern day diets is responsibile for the degeneration of our health. The reasons for this are simple. As a result of consuming imitation foods or nonfoods, we first undermine, and then destroy, our resistance to disease. Poor nutrition sets the stage for serious illness.

The information and recommendations in this chapter offer new hope and promise for those who already have cancer, and a simple plan of prevention to avoid contracting it in the first place. This is not just another "eat natural foods and everything will be all right" diet. It is scientifically based and clinically proven. The Livingston Anti-Cancer Diet, faithfully adhered to, can provide a longer, happier life, one with greater chances of being cancer-free.

In primitive societies man was forced to subsist on whatever food was available. Sometimes food was plentiful, sometimes scarce. When the primitive individual became incapacitated for any reason, he succumbed rapidly unless his illness was a short, self-limiting affliction. Our present society has the knowledge and skill to avert or shorten the onslaught of many serious, incapacitating diseases. We have turned to surgery and lifesaving drugs, such as antibiotics, to lengthen our life span. However, there are simpler things that nature has provided, which we, when properly informed and motivated, can use to prevent disease, alleviate ill health, and prolong life. These are the foods that we must learn to like and eat habitually as well as cultivating other personal habits such as avoidance of noxious substances (like alcohol and tobacco) and stressful personal habits. Most importantly, we can and should become educated in the simple principles of good nutrition. In a society commercially oriented toward the profit system, the mass production of cheap food, the use of preservatives to prolong shelf life, the exploitation of taste over quality, and convenience and attractive packaging, can lose unsuspecting consumers in a jungle of incomprehension, leading to general deterioration of their health and that of their offspring. Only the well informed can hope to avoid the nutritional pitfalls of such a society.

We have to start with the role of food in our life cycle. To begin with, our intestinal contents are our internal ecology. We are very particular about walking through mud puddles or contaminating our clothes and bodies, but we are not as selective about eating. Frequently, the intestinal tract is the American Garbage Can because of what we eat: foods that are infectious and foods that are badly balanced and lacking in nutrients. The results of what you eat may remain in your intestinal tract for a week, or even several weeks, as your body works to detoxify a chemical poison you happened to consume. The liver is the detoxifier and therefore under great stress. So when we talk about our intestinal tract and its functions, we are talking about an integral part of our entire life processes.

Our nutrition is dependent on our environment, the soil in which our food is grown, the animals that supply us with food-stuffs. When we eat the cells of infected animals, such as diseased cattle and cancerous chickens and eggs, their constituents become a part of us.

It is logical then that we cannot be perfectly healthy until we change this entire dietary approach, i.e., *clean up our diets.* Living plant food contains all the essentials for good health. If it is unprocessed, it can heal the body. When it is processed and altered, the essential factors are destroyed, rendering it useless.

Scientific evidence proving that a vegetarian diet is best for human beings is accumulating. Vegetables when raw or lightly cooked supply dietary enzymes and vitamins essential to good health that are not present in flesh foods. In addition, I reiterate that we've found that most of these flesh foods are highly con-taminated with pathogenic forms of the *P. Cryptocides* cancer-causing microbes (with some exceptions) and dangerous chem-icals, making them unfit for human consumption.

It may come as a shock to you that cattle are fed with chicken feces because the latter is rich in protein. The sick cattle are the ones that are sent to be slaughtered first. The sick chickens enter a race to either the frying pan or a hole in the ground.

After patients begin to recover, they are permitted selected fish and lamb. Only one sheep in a million develops cancer, perhaps because they eat primarily roots of plants, and roots are very high in abscisic acid. Shellfish are excluded from the diet because they are scavengers.

We all know the value of vitamin C in scurvy and the B vitamins in pellagra, but few of us know what other food factors can increase the restorative functions of the body when faced with serious disease. A person faced with a life-threatening disease such as cancer is usually willing to comply with any program that might prolong his or her life.

There are certain prohibitions, such as of cancer-infected foods, refined flour, white sugar, and empty calories devoid of vitamins and minerals. In their place we prescribe foods rich in minerals and vitamins and healing, nutritive substances. We have tried to present food that is palatable, adapted to the digestive capabilities of the sick, readily available, inexpensive, and not too difficult to prepare. This diet is not intended as a treatment for cancer, but rather as a way of raising immunity and increasing the patient's resistance to disease. The immune system can only be stimulated when the essential nutrients are available.

In addition to providing supplemental vitamins and minerals we are interested in presenting natural sources of the protective foodstuffs. We know that vitamin A guards against chemical carcinogenesis; vitamin C promotes healing; nicotinamide, B12, and riboflavin increase cellular oxidation; and abscisic acid neutralizes choriogonadotropin (the hormone which promotes the growth of cancer cells). All we ask is that each person study and read as much as possible to increase their knowledge and understanding of nutrition and health.

Before we get into the actual diet, let's look at a study by Dr. Weston A. Price, D.D.S., which investigated physical degeneration as related to diet. The following information is taken from Dr. Price's *Nutrition and Physical Degeneration* and concerns his studies of an isolated primitive culture in the Torres Strait Islands. He states, "It would be difficult to find a more happy and contented people than the primitives in the Torres Strait Islands as they lived without contact with modern civilization. They not only have nearly perfect bodies, but an associated personality and character of high excellence." He goes on to say that "in their native state they have exceedingly little disease. Dr. J. R. Nimmo, the government physician in charge of the supervision of this group, told me that in his thirteen years with them he had not seen a single case of malignancy, and had seen only one that he had suspected *might* be malignancy among the entire four thousand native population. He stated that during this same period he had operated on several dozen malignancies for the white population which numbered about three hundred."

Dr. Price's research showed definite evidence that degeneration had "an apparent direct relationship to the length of time government stores with civilized foods had been established." He stated that the primitives, wherever they adopted the white man's foods, "suffered the typical expressions of degeneration such as loss of immunity to dental decay and a marked lowering of resistance to disease."

As there is no single essential food, one of the most important goals of good nutrition is to be aware that whole foods, nearest to their natural state, are best able to supply the essential nutrients for the highest state of well-being. The following sixteen points from Dr. Price's findings should be the backbone of any good nutritional program:

1. In general, all the native foods were found to contain two to six times as high a factor of safety in the matter of body-building materials as did the displacing foods.

2. Minerals and fat soluble vitamins, from high vitamin butter, seafoods, cod liver oil, or seal oil, were consumed by nearly all groups studied.

3. All foods were grown on a highly mineralized soil with considerable humus content and no chemical fertilizers or pesticides.

4. All food was eaten liberally in the natural season.

5. Sweets (even natural ones) were used in moderation, usually only for occasions of ritual, celebration, or special feasting.

6. In each diet plan there was some regular source of unaltered raw protein, such as nuts and vegetables. (The essential amino acids must be included in the food choices for each meal or it will be impossible to assimilate the total values of the incomplete proteins. Learn to pay attention to balancing the amino acid patterns when vegetable proteins are eaten.)

7. Some sort of sea plant, animal or mineral, was part of every diet. Inland sea deposits of minerals were carefully used.

8. All nuts, grains, seeds, and fruits were eaten with their whole kernels. Dairy products were high in protective substances because the cattle ate grasses, grains, and seeds rich in nutritive elements.

9. The only methods of food preservation and storage used altered the nutrients very little (e.g., earth storage, drying, freezing in cold climates).

10. Each life style was such that all the people engaged in vigorous physical exercise on a regular basis, either by work or play, dances, games, or sports.

11. All had access to pure air and sunlight. (Even in the 1930s, Dr. Price realized the problems of air pollution and the lack of sufficient radiant energy from the sun due to the pollution already present at that time. Compare the pollution then with what is present today, and you have one explanation for the deterioration of our food quality and, as a result, our health.)

12. All of the primitives were able to instruct their young in these important principles, thereby protecting their genetic heritage. They ate the foods of their ancestors.

13. They all breast-fed their young.

14. Most of them fed special protective foods to their young people of childbearing age in preparation for conception, pregnancy, and lactation. Most of them had means of spacing the children at least three years apart to protect the children and their mothers.

15. They ate *whole* foods, not fractionalized parts of foods. They did not remove, by refining or otherwise, the valuable fiber content of their natural foods.

16. Most of their foods were eaten raw or very gently and lightly cooked.

These points are from my booklet, *Food Alive* (The Livingston-Wheeler Medical Clinic, 1975); and taken from Dr. Weston A. Price's *Nutrition and Physical Degeneration* (Price-Pottenger Foundation, Inc., N.D.).

It is obvious from this landmark study that not only do we have to change *what* we eat, but *how we prepare it.* Many people say, "I can get all the vitamins and minerals I need from a well-balanced diet." The problem is: "Balance" is no substitute for nutrients, and nutrients are becoming harder and harder to get from the average American meal.

On its way "from the garden to the gullet," chances are the food on your table has lost 50 percent or more of its important nutrients. Dr. Emanuel Cheraskin, of the University of Alabama School of Medicine and one of the greats in nutrition pioneering for the past thirty years, recently did a landmark study of a "typical well-balanced meal" of pork chops, potato, and vegetables. Here is how that meal gets nutritionally "mugged" on its way to your plate.

To begin with, food derives its nutritional strength from the soil it's grown in. The mineral content of much of the nation's arable land has been vastly reduced over the past 200 years, especially because of poisoning with pesticides and chemicals. When crops are ready for harvesting we may safely say that about 10 percent of their nutritional value has been lost. (The modern methods of feeding livestock are equally devastating to our meat products.)

During the time it takes to transport them to the store, fruits and vegetables have lost about 10 percent of their micronutrient value. This leaves you with 80 percent nutritional value on your plate.

What about the lengthy storage in the store once the food gets there? Especially in meats and vegetables, this can take another 10 percent out of the food. Now you have 70 percent for your meal.

An enormous amount of the food we eat, including our meat and vegetables, has been frozen somewhere along the line—either in a railroad car or in the store itself. And then *you* keep it frozen even longer in your refrigerator. Food can lose another

10 percent of its nutrients in the defrosting process—this leaves you with 60 percent.

Washing food, which is necessary because of surface contaminants, removes many minerals and vitamins that are most abundant on the skins and outer layers of fruits and vegetables. Let's say this loses another 5 percent, leaving you now with 55 percent.

Now consider how you prepare the food. Boiling, baking, and overcooking foods greatly reduce nutritional value. As much as 50 percent of the nutrients in vegetables are removed by the standard methods of cooking (especially overboiling). Conservatively, though, you probably boiled, broiled, baked, or sauteed about 20 percent of the nutrients out of the food you prepare. You now have about 35 percent—roughly *one-third*—of the nutrients on your dinner plate that you thought you had.

Now consider these: insecticides on your fruit; preservatives to keep your bread "fresh"; additives to make your beets redder; additives used in processing your cheese; sweeteners, such as those put into your catsup. The chemical reactions of these agents with the remaining nutrients in your food can render the vitamins and minerals inert. Often, you may not have any nutrients *at all* on your dinner plate, but let's say another 10 percent has been taken away by these unseen robbers.

You are now eating a meal with only 25 percent of the nutrients nature intended for you. A well-balanced meal? You'd have to eat *four times* that much to get what you thought you were getting.

It's not easy to *eat healthy*, but with a little extra effort it can be done. Here are some simple cooking Do's and Don'ts:

■ Methods of cooking that expose the food to hot grease, hot dry air, excessive heat, or smoke, such as frying, broiling, charcoal broiling, or oven roasting, and that produce a browning are to be avoided. This browning is an oxidative chemical reaction, and it produces toxins that have been reported to be carcinogenic, as well as fatty waste that causes a loss of nutritional value.

■ In addition to being subject to the effects of overheating and browning, charcoal broiled foods soak up the toxic fumes from the charcoal plus the fumes of the dripping burned grease.

■ Pressure cooking requires too high a temperature and may destroy valuable food elements.

■ Aluminum cookware reacts with certain foods, so we suggest that you avoid its use.

■ Electronic ovens are not recommended. Although cooking time is short, the excessive heat destroys valuable nutrients such as abscisic acid (which is destroyed at 275°F.) It is also said that essential sulfhydril groups are destroyed. Further investigation is needed.

The cooking Do's are simple. Use the least amount of water possible. (Waterless cooking is done in a stainless steel or ceramic steamer.) Prepare food as close to the time of eating as possible, as a time lapse between preparation and eating allows for oxidation, which can rob your food of valuable nutrients. Use the smallest amount of heat that will do the job. Each degree of temperature removes something of value.

A few things need to be said about kitchen equipment. Probably the most important piece of kitchen equipment required for your diet is a juicer, either a triturator or press kind. The triturator macerates the fruit or vegetable with the least amount of oxygenation, and the press separates the juice from the pulp. (Centrifugal juicers are not recommended because of oxidation of the juices.) Many of the pressure juicers will also grind grains, flour, and nuts.

A mini mill, such as a nut mill, coffee mill, or seed mill, is another invaluable piece of equipment. Basically, it consists of a small motorized or hand crank blade covered by a ½-cup container. It will grind nuts, seeds, and grains and costs only about twenty dollars.

Food graters and food processors are excellent investments and should be used to grate fruits and vegetables for sauces and salads.

Use only enamelware, stainless steel, Corningware, and Pyrex for cooking. They will not alter or detract from the nutritive value of the food. Crock pots are useful for legumes, but should not be used for other vegetables, as prolonged heating will destroy their nutrients. Waterless cookware, which requires a very small amount of water to cook the food, is very good. The heat is turned to medium until the lid rattles and then turned to as low a setting as possible for the remaining cooking time. All the vitamins and minerals in a food are retained. Ceramic or ironstone steamers or stainless steel steaming baskets are also useful; the vegetables are gently cooked by the steam, and flavor and nutritional substances also are retained.

ABSCISIC ACID

While not technically a vitamin, but rather an analog of vitamin A, nature's most potent anti-cancer weapon is abscisic acid. This is the essential immune ingredient which exists in nature as a portion of the vitamin A molecule. Hence it deserves special mention here before we discuss vitamin A itself.

Abscisic acid is the keystone upon which all cancer immunity is built in your body. If you already have cancer, abscisic acid is absolutely critical to your defense, because *abscisic acid actually stops cancer cells from multiplying.* If you don't have cancer (or if it is latent in your system), it is imperative that your diet contain high amounts of vitamin A and abscisic acid if you are to immunize yourself against it.

We universally find a low level of abscisic acid in all the patients who enter our clinic. You may have never heard of this unusual-sounding compound, but you can be sure that in the near future it will become as well known as vitamin C. In fact, abscisic acid is so important that I have been granted a use patent covering its anti-cancer effects.

The Livingston Anti-Cancer Diet naturally contains large amounts of vitamin A. The best foods for this vitamin are the yellow vegetables and certain fruits. The green leaves of vegetables are also very high in vitamin A, as are carrots. However, you will only get about one or two percent of the vitamin A in carrots when they are cooked. By making raw carrot juice, preferably in a juicer, you receive the benefits of *almost 100 percent* of the vitamin A.

But simply consuming large amounts of vitamin A is generally not enough. Certain malnourished people, and nearly all cancer patients, have lost the ability to break down vitamin A in their livers and make the essential abscisic acid. For these individuals I have included a table of foods which are high in abscisins. An even more effective way to increase the amount of abscisic acid in the diet is by treating carrot juice, for example, with liver powder (one heaping teaspoon to an 8 ounce glass of carrot juice). This is a low temperature dried liver powder from cancer free cattle that we use. When you add this powder, the liver enzymes in it form abscisic acid for you in the juice before you drink it. The powder does all the work for your liver. This is an excellent solution for cancer patients and healthy individuals alike; it's the easiest way to get the maximum benefits of this potent anti-cancer weapon.

Unfortunately, abscisic acid is not yet available for everyone to take as a daily supplement, although I hope it soon will be. If you were to purchase abscisic acid today, you would find that it costs approximately two hundred dollars per gram (there are 453 grams in a pound). However, by drinking carrot juice treated as I recommend, you can get six to eight grams from about a quart of carrot juice.

There has been a lot of recent research showing that vitamin A is very protective against the onset of cancer from carcinogens. Just in April of 1983, two articles appeared in *Lancet* and *The New England Journal of Medicine* reporting beneficial effects of retinoids (i.e., retinoic acids) in treating some bone and skin cancers. There is a group of vitamin A analogs that are classified as retinoids. Abscisic acid, the plant hormone called dormin, is a very important member of this class. This plant hormone is what causes seedlings to "go to sleep" in the autumn of the year. It actually suppresses plant growth. My research in the early days into what makes the cancer microbe grow made me want to find out what caused it to be suppressed. I suspected plant dormin might be the answer. (I was also a botanist in my premedical days at Vassar.)

I obtained a supply of this hormone from a pharmaceutical company and gave it to our infected lab animals. To my great joy, the abscisins (dormins) *did* inhibit the tumors. At the time, in the 1960s, I thought dormin was strictly a plant hormone, but, as it turns out, it is essential to our own lives as well as plants.

Our abscisic acid comes from the liver. Our livers break down vitamin A into the retinoids, which in turn have a large control over the choriogonadotropins (CG secretions) and cancer microbes. If you do not have the retinoic acids, you cannot build immunity. It's as simple as that.

Since vitamin A is destroyed by heat (abscisins in food are destroyed at only 275° F.), most food preparation methods leave our foods bankrupt of abscisic acid value. Even when the vitamin A and the abscisins are retained in your food, the condition of your liver determines how effectively your body can use them to build your immunity. If your liver is damaged for whatever reason—ingestion of chemicals from food contaminants, alcohol, disease, drugs, etc.—your liver enzymes are defective and unable to break down the vitamin A into retinoic acids.

Our experiments with mice have shown the beneficial anti-cancer effect of abscisic acid. When abscisic acid is given to mice after tumor implantation, and they have been preventatively immunized with the *P. Cryptocides* vaccine in one form or another, the tumors do not develop and kill the mice. The result of the experiment is an 80 to 90 percent rate of protection of the mice against the experimental implanted tumors. In contrast, when the mouse chow is sterilized by heat at a high temperature, such as by autoclaving (high temperature steam under pressure), the abscisins are destroyed and immunity does not develop unless fresh food is added. Many experiments in immunology fail because this action is not recognized.

Foods Containing Abscisic Acid

Fruits

Mangoes
Grapes
Avocados
Pears
Oranges with the white
    underpeel and pulp
Apples, whole with the seeds
Strawberries

Fruit blossoms
    and leaves as tea

Peach flowers
Strawberry leaves
Cherry flowers
Apple blossoms

Leafy vegetables

Mature Greens

Vegetables

Pea shoots
Lima beans
Potatoes
Dwarf peas
Yams
Sweet potatoes
Asparagus
Tomatoes
Onions
Spinach

Root vegetables

All root vegetables—
    especially carrots
(refer to shopping list)

Seeds and nuts

*All seeds, nuts, fruits, and fresh vegetables with their mature greens seem to contain abscisins.

GENERAL DIETARY INSTRUCTIONS
FOR CANCER PATIENTS

1. During the day fresh juices and homemade soups should be taken when thirsty instead of water. This helps to saturate the system with organically-combined minerals, vitamins, and live-oxidizing enzymes, aiding detoxification of the body. The exception to this suggestion is when nothing can be kept in the stomach and only water is retained.

2. Don't use fluoridated water for drinking or cooking. It is a cumulative enzyme poison, and cooking concentrates the fluoride. Read labels to make sure.

3. Food should be cooked in stainless-steel, waterless cookware: ironstone steamers, stainless steel steaming baskets, or vapor cookers. Avoid the use of pressure cookers, microwave ovens, or aluminum pots and utensils.

4. Do not drink alcoholic beverages or soft drinks. Also avoid iced drinks, as they inhibit and retard digestion.

5. Do not smoke or be in a room constantly with a smoker.

6. Don't eat refined or processed foods. The less refined and more primitive the diet, the better.

7. Eat organically grown, unsprayed, and unfumigated fruits and vegetables when available, or grow them yourself. The soil is your external metabolism. Home gardens with compost, earthworms, and natural fertilizers are important for your new way of life.

8. Wilted, pale, flabby, soft-spotted, imperfect fruits and vegetables rob you of vitality and building nutrients.

9. Use a biodegradable detergent with a vegetable base for your dishwashing, laundry, and produce washing. One-quarter teaspoon to 1 gallon of water is a good solution, and after using, discard it in the garden—it will be well utilized!

10. When gas bloat and indigestion occur immediately after eating, it may be an indication of a lack of HCL in the stomach. To help alleviate the condition, HCL tablets or Dil. HCL should be used with meals. The amount taken

will depend on the acidity of the urine as indicated by Nitrazine paper.

11. Increase the potassium foods such as greens, potatoes, lima beans, nuts, and most fruits and vegetables.

12. Decrease the high sodium foods, which include most processed salted foods.

13. Become a label detective. Read *all* labels. Avoid artificial colors, flavors, preservatives, and sugar substitutes. Watch out for preservatives such as BHT and BHA, even when used in the containers.

14. Get at least eight hours of sleep, plus regular relaxation periods. Exercise daily according to your ability and, if possible, outside in the sun. Sunbathing may also be beneficial. Take hot baths daily to increase circulation. Cultivate a positive mental attitude.

15. Avoid permanent wave solutions and hair colors, toxic hair sprays, synthetic cosmetics, and especially lipsticks made out of coal tar dyes and antiperspirants with aluminum ingredients. Try lemon juice or acidophilus under your arms as a deodorant. Use natural cosmetics. Use only non-allergenic *natural* deodorants. Do not feed your hair and skin these poisonous chemicals. Avoid cleaning solutions, solvents, paint removers, and insect sprays.

16. Learn to substitute: arrowroot for thickening; yeast/power-beater for leavening instead of eggs; oil and butter instead of shortening; and nut or seed milk for cow's milk. Use soy milk if desired and whipping cream, raw if possible; Cellu low sodium baking powder or yeast for baking powder; kelp or vegetable herb seasoning for salt.

17. Add one heaping teaspoon of ascorbic acid powder to juices, soups, teas as tolerated.

18. Add nuts to any recipe to increase the protein content, choosing the nuts that you most enjoy.

19. Limit yourself to one or two pieces of citrus fruit per day because of the high sugar content, and eat whole except for the skin (as opposed to juicing).

20. Milk may be used in limited quantities for the recovered patient and only on physician recommendation. A limited quantity would be eight ounces per day of raw, certified milk which is better since it has a lower bacterial count than regular milk.

21. Try to combine legumes, grains, and leafy vegetables in planning your individual meals. For example, in the Republic of China the government-recommended diet for men performing heavy labor is as follows:

500 grams	Leafy green vegetables
500 grams	Cereal
60 grams	Soybean
400 grams	Sweet potato

This ration combines the grain, the legume, the leafy green vegetables, and the natural sweet.

22. At most, 1–2 dates or figs per day are allowed.

23. Read labels on products used for sweetening to make sure they contain no artificial sweeteners.

24. Use any good vegetable seasoning, such as Savorex or Dr. Bronner's Soup Mix, interchangeably in all recipes.

25. Carrot sticks, celery and other raw vegetables, nuts, and dried foods are excellent snacks.

FOODS TO AVOID

Beverages	Alcohol, cocoa, coffee, milk, soft drinks.
Bread	White bread and blended breads made out of white flour.
Cereals	Processed cereals are puffed and sugared. No white rice.
Cheese	Only as directed when recovered.
Desserts	Canned or frozen fruits. All pastries, gelatin, custards, sauces, ice cream, candy, except those made of suggested health ingredients.

Eggs	Forbidden from unvaccinated chickens. Use Jolly Joan Egg Replacer.
Fat	Shortening, margarine, saturated oils and fats. Rancid and continuously heated oils.
Fish	Smoked and salted fish. Fish preserved in antibiotics. No shellfish.
Fruits	Sprayed and sulfured. Canned and frozen.
Juices	All canned and frozen juices except frozen pineapple juice.
Meats	*No unvaccinated poultry*. *No pork* in any form, or fat such as bacon, ham, or ribs. No fried, smoked, salted, or processed meats such as sausages and cold cuts. No beef or veal.
Milk	Whipping cream and raw butter (if available) may be used in moderation.
Nuts	Salted nuts.
Potatoes	French fries, potato chips.
Soups	Canned or frozen soup, fat stock, bouillion, dehydrated consomme.
Sprouts	Mature sprouts.
Sweets	White sugar and white sugar products such as candy, all sugar substitutes, and honey except as directed.
Vegetables	Sprayed, canned. Sulfur and high sodium foods. Frozen vegetables preferable to canned when fresh not available.

AVOID ALL CHEMICALS, CLEANING SOLUTIONS, SOLVENTS, PAINT REMOVERS, INSECT SPRAYS, DEODORANTS, HAIR DYES, DISINFECTANTS, PEST STRIPS, ETC.

FOODS TO INCLUDE

Avocado	Mash ¼ avocado with a fork and stir into each glass of freshly pressed juice. Allow it to remain 15–20 minutes.

Beverages	Herb teas, sesame or nut milk, soy milk, cereal beverages (such as Postum), dandelion or chicory teas.
Breads	Millet, rye, buckwheat, whole wheat, bran, corn, seven-grain, corn tortillas. Only whole grains— freshly ground and free of all preservatives. The abscisins are lost in sprouted grain bread if baked over 300°F.
Cereals	Millet, oatmeal, brown and wild rice, buck-wheat, alfalfa, groats, barley, cornmeal, oatmeal, cracked wheat, and seven-grain. Freshly ground rolled flakes or whole grain only.
Cheese	Only as directed and not until recovered.
Desserts	Fresh, whole fruits, fresh fruit cocktails, natural fruit gelatin, health desserts and snacks made of outlined ingredients.
Fat	Olive oil, avocados, butter (raw if possible), and sesame oil.
Fish	Fresh water and sea fish, broiled, baked, or poached. Avoid polluted shellfish.
Fruits	Fresh fruits, organically grown if possible. Apples, apricots, bananas, berries, cherries, currants, grapes, guava, mangoes, melon, nectarines, papaya, peaches, pineapple, pears, plums, persimmons, tangerines, unsulfured dried fruits— apples, apricots, figs, peaches, prunes. Where possible, eat the seeds or kernels with the fruit.
Juices	Only freshly pressed juices and frozen pineapple juice. The pressed juices may be selected from the list of fruits and vegetables listed. Apple and carrot are the most popular. Include mature beet leaves, chicory, escarole, Swiss chard, watercress, beets, cucumber.
Meat	Lamb and its internal organs. Lamb heart and extra fresh lamb liver are permitted.
Milk	Substitute: soy milk, seed and nut milks such as sesame, sunflower, almond, and cashew.

Nuts   Fresh, raw nuts, particularly walnuts, almonds, cashews, pecans, peanuts, and apricot pits. Raw nut butters, freshly made in the blender or juicer only.

Potatoes   Baked or steamed with jackets. Sweet potatoes are an important dietary addition. Substitute: millet, brown rice, wild rice, occasional noodles made with the flour of buckwheat, whole wheat, soya, or artichoke. Use those noodles made without eggs, and *avoid* white flour!

Salads   Use raw fruits and mature vegetables listed. Shredded or chopped, separate or combined, such as shredded apple and carrot.

Seasoning   Chives, garlic, parsley. Herbs: laurel, marjoram, sage, thyme, savory, kelp, vegetable and herb seasonings without sodium chloride (table salt). Dr. Bernard Jensen's vegetable broth and seasoning is very good. Sea salt is permitted in limited amounts. Savorex natural lemon juice.

Seeds   Sunflower, flax, sesame, and pumpkin—fresh and raw.

Soups   Homemade soups made from listed ingredients. Barley, brown rice, or millet can be added.

Sprouts   Sprouts to the age of eight days are permitted since vitamin A and the abscisins are very rich in these, but after eight days the gibberellins are produced, which promote rapid growth of seedlings and tumors and neutralize the abscisic acid.

Sweets   Use only ½ tsp. of honey on Diets 2 and 3 and even less, if any, on Diet 1.

Vegetables   Organically grown raw or freshly cooked. Artichokes, asparagus, beets, broccoli, carrots, cauliflower, chives, corn, endive, green and wax beans, kale, legumes, potatoes, spinach, squash, Swiss chard, watercress, and any fresh seasonal vegetable.

RECOMMENDED SUBSTITUTES

Foods Not to Use	Substitutes
Sugar Honey Molasses Maple syrup Date sugar	Carrot, apple, papaya, or pineapple juice will provide enzymes and sweetness, if necessary. A new sweetener from grapefruit is available as a substitute for the artificial coal tar sweeteners.
Chocolate	Carob

Hydrogenated fats
  (lard, shortening,
  etc.)
	Unsaturated oils:
	Olive oil, sesame oil, raw butter (if possible) in small amounts.
	Untreated cold pressed oils.

White flour	Flours made from whole grains, nuts, seeds. Grind fresh yourself: rye, corn, millet, barley, buckwheat, sunflower seed, brown rice, oat, whole wheat. Soy flour may be purchased.
Whole milk	Whipping cream (raw if possible and may add lemon juice), soy milk from soybean, soy milk from soy flour reconstituted with water, nut and seed milks.
Thickening agents	Brown wheat flour Arrowroot Brown rice flour Soy flour or rye flour

Commercial
  leavening agents
  (baking powder or
  soda)
	Yeast

Eggs	Egg replacers
Salt (table salt)	Kelp, sea salt, sesame salt

12
MENUS
AND
RECIPES

OUR DIETS AT THE CLINIC are divided into three separate diet plans, according to the condition of the patient. Patients who are extremely ill and often nauseated are given vegetable juices, primarily because they are easy to take and most immediately beneficial. For the patients who cannot even tolerate vegetable juices, a tablespoon of grain meal water added to the glass of juice has been found to be soothing to the gastrointestinal tract and aids in containing the nausea.

As soon as the patient is able, we then add about one-quarter of a ripe avocado to the juice. This is done by simply mashing the avocado with a fork or spoon and stirring it in. The avocado helps break down the carotene in the carrot juice into vitamin A analogs. Avocados are excellent sources of abscisins.

The next food to add to the diet is usually Basic Muesli (see page 173). Since it's very easy on the digestive system, it may be prepared in a variety of ways and used as a basic breakfast food or a snack during the day.

As the patient progresses, both raw and cooked soups are added and then whole grain cereals freshly ground in a mini mill. The patient may then be ready to try whole grain breads. Abscisins are high in plants that are ready to flower, such as the green tips of broccoli, etc., and in sprouted seedlings not over seven days old.

We also advise patients not to drink large amounts of water, so that the maximum amounts of raw vegetable juices can be consumed.

At the clinic we have Diet #1 for *acutely ill* cancer patients. Diet #2 is for *recuperating* patients, i.e., those who have started to improve. Diet #3 is for the patient on a *maintenance* program, i.e., the patient who is on the road to recovery. This diet is also good for those people who want to change their diet habits completely in order to promote immunity.

It is important to remember that at least 50 percent of the food must be raw. Some patients have stayed on totally raw food for one year or more.

A word about strict diets. It is awfully hard to maintain very strict diets such as this one in modern day America. I fully realize that some people are lazy, tend toward self-indulgence, and avoid things that "aren't any fun." We have had several acutely ill patients at the clinic who simply refused to give up smoking, drinking, meat, chicken and eggs, and they have not progressed as they should.

Healthy people, especially, have a hard time changing their diet patterns. A healthy person doesn't want to give up alcohol, or smoking, or any of a dozen other things, *until he or she gets sick*. Once a person is told she has cancer of the breast with metastases, it becomes exceptionally easy to do anything to change the course of the disease. A man with cancer of the lung will quit smoking immediately. In other words, you knew you would die tomorrow if you had one more drink, you would quit drinking. If you knew the *very next* cigarette would give you lung cancer, you wouldn't light up.

So, of course our diets look exceedingly strict. But they only look strict to the healthy reader. To a person dying of cancer, they seem to be blessedly easy to follow.

For the purpose of this book we have included menus for a strict and a non-strict diet, only.

I. STRICT DIET

	Recommended Items	Forbidden Items
Beverages	Fresh vegetable juices. Carrot up to 1 quart/day. Fresh juices. Chamomile tea, mint tea, papaya tea, rose hip tea, other herb teas.	Alcohol, cocoa, coffee, milk, soft drinks.
Bread	WHOLE GRAIN—rye bread, whole wheat or bran muffins, whole wheat bread or homemade bread from recipes given.	Any other commercial breads. NO WHITE BREAD.
Cereals	WHOLE GRAIN UNPROCESSED buckwheat, cornmeal, cracked wheat, millet, oatmeal, sesame, fine ground grits, whole grain sprouted grains up to seven days of sprouting.	All other. Refined and bleached flour. White rice.
Cheese	NONE	All forbidden.
Dessert	Fresh fruits: three per day.	Custards, junkets, all pastries, puddings sauces, and ice creams.
Eggs	NONE—use Jolly Joan Egg Replacer.	In any form.
Fat	Olive oil, butter, sesame oil	Shortening, margarine, saturated oils and fats.
Fruits	FRESH ONLY: apples, pears, apricots, bananas, cherries, currants, grapes, guava, mangoes, melon, nectarines, papaya, peaches, plums, ripe oranges, quince, ripe pineapple, avocados.	Canned fruits. Dried fruits (unsulfured) should be used in moderation, as they do contain sugar and are not fresh.
Juices	ONLY FRESH JUICES. May be selected from lists of fruits and vegetables permitted, including the following green leaves: mature beet leaves, broccoli, chicory, endive, escarole, lettuce, Swiss chard, and watercress. Carrot will be used most often. One whole orange per day, but fruit juices may be too high in sugar.	All canned juices, juices with artificial coloring and sweetening.

Meat	NONE NO POULTRY	No pork, fat, fried and smoked meat, or sausages; no chicken or turkey.
Milk	Whipping cream, soy milk, nut milk and seed milks.	Dairy products.
Nuts	All types of fresh, raw nuts; almonds, 6 to 10 a day with whole apple. Cashews are excellent.	Roasted and salted nuts and peanuts.
Potatoes	Baked, boiled. Potato salad made with homemade eggless mayonnaise.	French fries, chips.
Salads	The following raw vegetables shredded or finely chopped, separated or mixed: carrots, cauliflower, celery, chicory, bell peppers, tomatoes, watercress, turnips, parsnips, broccoli, lettuce, radishes, Swiss chard, asparagus, artichokes (Jerusalem), cabbage, mushrooms, beets, squashes.	
Seasoning	Chives, garlic, onion, parsley, herbs, laurel, marjoram, sage, thyme, savory, cumin, oregano, sea salt, kelp, papaya seed pepper, sesame salt.	Hot spices, pepper, sodium salt.
Soups	HOMEMADE—vegetable soup; barley, millet, brown or wild rice may be added. Raw vegetable soups are especially recommended such as gazpacho.	All canned consommé and soups including dehydrated. NO fat stock.
Vegetables	RAW OR FRESHLY COOKED: artichokes, asparagus, carrots, cauliflower, celery, chives, corn, endives, green leeks, spinach, green peas, bell peppers, leeks, lentils, lima beans, potatoes, radishes, tomatoes, wax beans, yams, eggplant, squash, sweet potatoes. Any vegetables listed under salads. All seasonal vegetables.	Sprayed, canned or frozen.

STRICT DIET
SUGGESTED MENUS

Menu #1

BREAKFAST

8-oz. glass carrot juice containing ¼ avocado
Basic Millet with Nut Cream
Whole grain toast, if desired
Violet leaf tea
Supplements, as prescribed

LUNCH

Grated carrot with
    Garden Salad Supreme,
    Horseradish Dressing
Black Bean Soup
Curried Vegetables
Vegetable snack: choice of
    squash, okra, zucchini, celery,
    carrots, turnip and parsnip (raw)
Whole grain bread and butter
Strawberry leaf tea
Supplements, as prescribed

DINNER

Garden Salad Supreme
Cream of Mushroom Soup
Spaghetti Squash
Whole grain bread and butter
Peppermint leaf tea
Supplements, as prescribed

SNACKS

Mid-morning
Fresh vegetable juice or fresh fruit
Whole grain bread and butter

Mid-afternoon
Fresh vegetable juice or fresh fruit. (If hungry, use tahini
   over fruit or on toast.)

Evening
Fresh vegetable juice
Nuts or seeds
Raw vegetable soup

Menu #2

BREAKFAST

8-oz. glass of carrot juice with ¼ avocado
Basic Muesli served with Nut Cream or whipping cream
Strawberry leaf tea
Toasted whole grain bread and butter, if still hungry

LUNCH

Artichoke Salad with Lemon and Oil Dressing
Cream of Vegetable Soup
Baked potato with raw butter
Lentils and Onions
   (If still hungry, add raw carrots, celery, pepper strips
   or any gently steamed vegetable.)
Whole grain bread and butter
Herb tea of choice

DINNER

Grated carrots with Horseradish Dressing
Raw Avocado Tomato Soup
Herbed Millet
Steamed asparagus with Eggless Mayonnaise II
Whole grain bread and butter
Herb tea of choice
Take supplements with meals, as prescribed.

SUGGESTED SNACKS

Mid-morning
8-oz. glass of juice with ¼ avocado mashed with fork
  and stirred in
If still hungry, eat some cashew nuts.

Mid-afternoon
8 oz. fresh juice
Apple slices with tahini (sesame butter)

Evening
8 oz. fresh juice
7 almonds

NON-STRICT DIET SUGGESTED MENUS

One quart of mixed vegetable and carrot juice per day is recommended. The main meal of the day should be at midday. The
same snacks would apply as in the strict diet.

BREAKFAST

Glass of vegetable juice
Raw fruit
Porridge and seed milk or cream
Whole grain toast and butter
Herb tea
Supplements

LUNCH

Salad—large green leaves
Soup (raw or cooked)
Potato, rice, or bread
Main dish, such as legumes or nut loaf
Steamed vegetables
Whole grain bread and butter
Herb tea
Supplements

DINNER

Salad
Soup (raw)
Brown rice or millet
Vegetables, raw or lightly steamed
Whole grain bread and butter
Herb tea
Supplements

Shopping List

Before we begin preparing menus, it is essential that we have purchased the proper ingredients. Following is a shopping list of suggested foods to help you get started.

Fruits

papaya	oranges*	apricots
pears	mangoes*	grapefruits
apples	grapes*	tangerines
currants	strawberries*	melons*
	peaches*	bananas

*when in season or personally fresh frozen if necessary.

Vegetables

avocados	asparagus	artichokes:
carrots	corn	(Jerusalem
lima beans	spinach	and
tomatoes	beets	globe)
green onion	turnips	beet greens
celery	rutabagas	kale
potatoes	large lettuces,	mustard greens
sweet potatoes	Romaine	cabbage
comfrey	endives	cauliflower
turnip greens	parsley	chard
cucumbers	radishes	lentils
	kohlrabi	soy beans

Whole Grains
and Breads

wheat flakes	brown rice	millet
rye flakes	buckwheat	oats
bulgur	open pollinated	rye
barley	corn	triticale
		whole wheat

Bread Spreads

sesame tahini   all types nut butters

Nuts

hazelnuts   walnuts   macadamia nuts
almonds, 5 lbs.   pine nuts   pecans
cashews

Whenever possible nuts in shells are preferable. They become rancid when shelled and stored too long.

Seeds

sesame   flax   pumpkin
sunflower

Beverages

strawberry leaf tea   papaya mint tea   fresh ginger tea
red clover tea   fenugreek seed tea   flax tea
dandelion tea   peach blossom tea   Kaffree tea
peppermint tea   rose hip tea

Miscellaneous

Fearns Soy Powder   raw butter   Dr. Jensen's Broth
   or natural soy   raw cream   Seasoning
   powder   Savorex

RECIPES

BEVERAGES

When the very ill cannot tolerate anything but beverages, what they primarily need is vegetable juices. Because of this, the basis of this diet is raw vegetable juices, freshly extracted.

It is important to select the best quality of naturally grown produce that you can find. Be certain to wash the fruits and vegetables carefully, scrubbing with a vegetable brush and removing any bruised, wilted, or otherwise damaged parts.

The importance of clean, organically grown fruits and vegetables cannot be stressed enough, because chemically grown or pesticide-sprayed produce have poisons concentrated in their juices.

Be sure to follow carefully the instructions that come with your juice extractor, so that you do not inadvertently lose all the vitamins. Prepare your juices three times a day. *Do not* make juice ahead for the next meal, and *do not* store it any longer than two hours, or it will lose the vital nutrients your body so desperately needs. After partial recovery, the addition of 10 grams vitamin C to the juice will help to preserve its potency for several hours.

Remember, when drinking juices you are consuming many times the vegetables and fruits that you would were you eating them whole, so you are reaping multiple benefits from one glass of juice.

Carrot juice is used primarily, often in combination with other juices, because of its high abscisic content. It is suggested that juices be drunk instead of water when thirsty, so that nutritional benefits can be utilized by the body. If possible, drink at least one quart of carrot juice each day.

Juices

FRESH JUICES

Vegetables and fruits should be brushed and washed. Peel them only if it is necessary. A press-type juicer is preferred (less loss of nutrients through oxidation). Always drink juices freshly made, if possible. Do not add ice.

Quantity: At frequent intervals, according to the patient's reactions or as prescribed by the physician. Drink juices in addition to spring water.

The following combinations of juices
are suggested for variety:

3 parts carrot juice to 1 part apple juice;
3 parts carrot juice to 1 part spinach juice;
3 parts carrot juice to 1 part cabbage juice;
4 parts carrot juice, 2 parts cucumber juice, and
1 part beet juice;
1 part carrot juice to 3 parts fresh tomato juice;
Equal parts carrot and cucumber juice.

Herb Teas

Fruit tree blossoms, such as cherry, peach, and apple, contain abscisic acid, and if naturally grown and available, they can be brewed into delightful teas, but do not boil them. Or the blossoms may simply be added to other herb teas to enhance their flavors. Fresh blossoms are preferable, but they can be dried in a low temperature food dehydrator to extend their availability.

Rose hips, obtained from naturally grown rose bushes that have not been sprayed with insecticides, may be gathered, dried, and freshly ground to make a delicious herb tea. Many health food stores sell organically grown rose hip tea.

Other garden leaves that make delightful teas are strawberry and violet leaves, and a variety of herbs. Lemon leaves make a flavorful addition to herb teas. Other good additions to your herb tea are the peels from oranges, lemons, or tangerines, if they have not been sprayed or dyed. Dry them in your food dehydrator or in an oven that is heated only by the pilot light or light bulb, and then store the dried peel in a tightly covered jar. This crisp, flavorful rind, high in nutrients and bioflavanoids, is always ready to add to your herb teapot.

Experiment with herbal teas. Most health food stores have a good variety, and books on herbs can be purchased from most local bookstores or borrowed from your library. Be sure the herbs used are compatible with your condition.

For best results, pour hot water over the herbs and let the tea steep in a warm teapot. Avoid boiling to prevent denaturalization. Then sit back and enjoy new flavor treats with natural teas.

HERB TEA

¼ cup (tightly packed) garden-fresh herb leaves *or*
¼ to ½ cup dried herb leaves
1 quart water

If herbs are fresh, blend them in water, strain, and drink cold or gently warmed. If herbs are dried, place them in water, set them in the sun all day, refrigerating overnight.

Suggestion: Several handfuls of dried mint can be tossed into a large jar filled with water. Stir frequently, straining off and diluting as you need. The pitcher can be filled several times before the flavor is used.

Nut and Seed Milks

SOY MILK

Choose a full-fat soy bean powder for making soy milk, rather than a defatted powder, as vitamin A is in the fat part of the seed or bean.

Mix 1 cup of full-fat soy bean powder to 4 cups water. Let soak about 2 hours, mix again, and transfer to a double boiler to cook for 20 minutes. Strain through a fine sieve and use *only* one of the following for flavoring:

> ¼ cup carob powder
> 2 teaspoons vanilla
> 1 cup apple juice
> 1 cup unsweetened prune juice
> 1 cup papaya juice (reconstituted Hanson's)
> 1 cup carrot juice
> 1 tablespoon de-cyanided apricot pit meal
>   with 1 teaspoon vanilla

ALMOND MILK

> 1 cup almonds, ground
> 4 cups water

Blend for 2 minutes and add one of the following if you so desire: 1 teaspoon kelp *or* 2 tablespoons currants *or* several small dates, pitted.

APPLE ALMOND MILK

> ¼ cup almonds, ground
> 1½ cups apple juice, freshly juiced

Blend and chill. Do not keep overnight.

CARROT ALMOND MILK

1 cup carrot juice
½ cup almonds, ground
2 cups water

Place ground nuts in blender with water and blend for two minutes. Add one cup of almond milk to one cup carrot juice. Do not keep; use at once. Serves two.

Suggestion: This can be served as a soup, also. (Warmed or cool.)

SUNFLOWER SEED MILK

1 cup sunflower seeds, ground
2 cups water
4 drops vanilla
¼ teaspoon kelp
1 tablespoon currants (optional)

Blend together 2 minutes, adding more water if desired.

CASHEW MILK

1 cup cashews
2 cups water
¼ teaspoon kelp (optional)

Blend all ingredients together for 2 minutes, using more water if desired. Serves 2.

NUT CREAM

1 tablespoon cashews, raw
1 tablespoon almonds, raw
1 tablespoon sesame seeds, raw
¾ cup water

1½ tablespoons coconut juice
¼ teaspoon vanilla
½ teaspoon honey, raw

Grind the nuts and seeds until fine in the blender, and add the water on a high speed until well combined. Blend the nut milk with the remaining ingredients until smooth. Serve with breakfast cereals or fruit.

SESAME MILK

½ cup sesame seeds
2 cups water and 2 dates, pitted,
   or
dried fruit, soaked in water

Blend all the ingredients together and enjoy.

SESAME CREAM

½ cup sesame seeds
½ cup water
½ cup carrot juice
A few drops of vanilla (optional)

Blend together the sesame seeds and water until smooth. Add the carrot juice and vanilla, blending lightly.

Variation: A banana may be blended in instead of the carrot juice.

SESAME NUT CREAM

1 cup Sesame Milk, above
½ cup almond butter or cashew butter
2 dates, chopped and pitted

Blend well and serve over fruit or fruit salads.

GRAINS, GRAIN WATERS, CEREALS

Purchase *whole*, naturally grown grains only. A whole grain is fairly stable and can be stored for some time in quart glass jars with a few bay leaves to prevent infestation. Ground grains deteriorate and become rancid rapidly, causing the vitamin E in the grain germ to become damaged. Even refrigerated ground grain loses its nutrients in five days.

Included in the grain family are barley, buckwheat, corn, millet, oats, rice, rye, and wheat. You can grind ¼ cup at a time of any whole grain in your mini mill, but it is advisable to grind only as much as you will use at once. Grinding for a few seconds will produce a coarse cereal grind; longer grinding will give you flour.

The easiest way to prepare these whole grains is to stir 1 part whole grain into 2 parts boiling water and continue to boil for about 10 minutes. Then remove from the heat, cover, and let soak overnight. In the morning, reheat for a hot cereal or eat cold. Any remaining liquid can be used as a nutritious drink or added to recipes. Overnight sprouted grains warmed in the morning make an excellent, tasty cereal. Some grains may require rinsing and sprouting for two to three days before using.

Do not buy your cereal flakes at the supermarket. They are usually lacking in the essential nutrients you need for recovery.

Grain Waters

Grain waters are very easily assimilated and digested. They provide, therefore, gastrointestinal relief. Naturally grown whole grains should be freshly ground and used for these recipes. One tablespoon of any of the following recipes may be added to raw juices to neutralize the tart juice flavor.

They are to be used as a comfort food when you are not feeling well.

GRAIN MEAL WATER

**1 tablespoon of any whole grain or grain mixture
(freshly ground whole grain rye, rice, barley, or millet)
1 pint water**

Mix the ground grain or combination of grains with cold water. Bring to a boil and simmer over low heat for one hour. Cool and serve (as with all other grain waters) when needing a comforting food.

BARLEY WATER

May be prepared as the other grain water recipes or as follows:

**2 ounces whole barley
3 pints water**

Combine ingredients and boil until the quantity of water is reduced by half. A few figs or currants may be blended into the cooled mixture to provide flavoring and a more laxative nature.

RICE WATER

**1 heaping teaspoon rice ground in mini mill
1 cup water**

Mix ground rice with cold water. Bring to a boil. Cook 5 minutes, stirring constantly.

CORN MEAL WATER

**1 tablespoon naturally grown whole corn, freshly ground
1 pint water**

Mix the corn meal with cold water. Bring to a boil and simmer on low heat for one hour. Cool and use ⅛ cup or so with your juice if desired. It may also be used plain.

CREAM OF WHEAT WATER

1 tablespoon naturally grown whole
    wheat berries, freshly ground
1 pint water

Mix the ground wheat with cold water. Bring to a boil and simmer on low heat for one hour. Cool and serve when needing a comforting food.

Cereals

OATMEAL

2 cups water
½ teaspoon kelp
1 cup oatmeal (natural, not processed)

Bring water and kelp to a boil. Slowly stir in rolled oats until mixture returns to a boil. Lower heat to a simmer. Cover and cook 3 to 5 minutes more or until water is absorbed.

Note: Some people find oatmeal more digestible if it is boiled and soaked in water overnight and then heated in the morning.

BUCKWHEAT GROATS

¼ cup butter
½ cup mushrooms, ½ cup onions
    and/or green pepper (optional)
1 cup kasha or buckwheat groats
2 cups water

Melt butter in pan and sauté mushrooms, onions and green pepper if desired. Add buckwheat groats to mixture (or just to butter), and then add the water. Cover and steam 15 minutes on lowest heat. Serve with butter. Serves 4.

CREAM OF MILLET

¼ cup millet or other whole grain
1 cup water
1 teaspoon kelp
1 tablespoon currants

Grind the millet in a mill. Bring the water to a boil and add kelp and currants. Cover tightly and simmer for 5 minutes.

FLAXSEED AND CURRANT CEREAL

1 cup boiling water
½ cup coarsely ground flaxseed
1 teaspoon kelp
⅓ cup currants
¼ cup walnuts
1 teaspoon vanilla (optional)

Combine the flaxseed and hot water. Add the remaining ingredients, cover and let stand for five minutes. Serve with a nut milk, pages 164 and 165, or diluted raw cream.

BARLEY CEREAL

½ cup naturally grown whole barley
2 cups water

Combine the barley and water. Bring to a boil and simmer until barley is tender.

Currants may be added to provide flavor.

CREAM OF RICE CEREAL

4 cups brown rice
¼ cup tamari (natural soy sauce)
¾ cup water
Butter

Wash the rice well, and place it damp into a heavy skillet. Stir the rice while toasting until it becomes crisp and dry. Pour the rice into a bowl and mix in the tamari until all liquid is absorbed. Lay out on a towel to cool and dry. (Store extra in a glass jar. This makes a good snack food!) Grind ¼ cup of this rice in your mill. Add the ground rice to the water and simmer gently for 20 minutes. Add butter when ready to serve.

BASIC MILLET

2 cups water
1 teaspoon salt
1 teaspoon kelp
⅔ cup millet

Bring water to boil. Add remaining ingredients. Cover and simmer 20 minutes or more. Millet should be light and fluffy when properly cooked.

Millet is alkaline in nature and, for a cereal, considered high in protein.

BASIC BROWN RICE

1 cup brown rice
2 cups water
Vegetable broth and seasoning to taste
3 tablespoons sesame seeds, lightly toasted (optional)

Wash the rice. Bring the water and seasoning to a boil. Add rice, cover, and allow to simmer without stirring for 45 minutes. If sesame seeds are used, lightly toast them in a dry pan and add when the rice is finished.

BASIC WILD RICE

Wild rice is not a rice. It is a unique grain, *high in vitamins and protein. No one has been able to cultivate it successfully.*

⅔ cup wild rice
3 cups boiling water
½ teaspoon herb seasoned salt, or to taste
Butter (optional)

Wash the rice well. Pour the boiling water over the rice; cover and simmer until tender, approximately 45 minutes. Add the sea salt and butter, if desired. (Raw butter is superior, if available.) Serves 2.

BEST CEREAL

Any whole grain cereal may be prepared by stirring 1 cup of grain into 2 cups of boiling water, boiling 10 minutes, turning off the heat, and allowing it to sit overnight. It may also be poured into a wide mouth Thermos, which will keep it warm until breakfast time.

Any grain may be sprouted for 2 to 3 days, rinsing twice daily, then when sprouted, warmed and served as a cereal. Sprouted grains are more life invigorating than cooked. Chia, flax, sesame, and sunflower seeds soaked overnight make an excellent breakfast cereal when heated gently.

Other grains such as wheat, rye, and barley may require several days of sprouting.

We wish to utilize the abscisic acid present in the young plants and avoid gibberellic acid in older sprouts (7 days on) which promotes growth.

MUESLI

Muesli is a combination of finely grated (or chopped) fruit, soaked cereal flakes, ground seeds, and ground nuts. Mueslis are one of the best and tastiest ways to consume the seeds and grains that are highest in abscisins.

Preparation begins the evening before, starting with rolled cereal grains such as rolled oats, rye flakes, wheat flakes, millet, rice or barley flakes, or freshly ground whole grains. Purchase your fresh grain at a health food store—boxed cereals are not acceptable. The flakes or ground grains are soaked in pure water or pineapple juice for 8 to 12 hours. One-half tablespoon currants per serving may be soaked with the ground or flaked grains for added taste.

When ready to eat muesli, mix the measured amount of ground seeds or flaked grains with the freshly grated (or chopped) fruits in season: apples, apricots, peaches, strawberries, blueberries, blackberries, raspberries, plums, or other allowed fruits. Nuts are then freshly ground and served as the crowning glory to this delicious meal. Various recipe combinations follow.

BASIC MUESLI

 1 tablespoon rye flakes
 1 tablespoon oat flakes
 ¼ cup pure water or pineapple juice
 ½ tablespoon currants

Combine ingredients and soak overnight. Next morning, add:

 ¾ cup grated raw apple topped with
 1 tablespoon ground almonds

MUESLI VARIETY

 ½ tablespoon rye flakes
 ½ tablespoon rice flakes
 ½ tablespoon wheat flakes
 3 tablespoons water

Combine ingredients and soak overnight. Next morning, add:

 ½ to ¾ cups grated or chopped apple, topped with
  1 tablespoon ground nuts

Additional Nut Cream, page 165, may be added if desired.

BREAD

The only wholesome bread is that which is made from grains that have been ground into flour only a few hours before baking. To get such flour, you must purchase it from a supplier who grinds grain daily, or get a mill and grind your own. The grain should be high protein, grown on soil that has not been depleted but organically fertilized. Such grain may cost you twice as much as lower quality, but it is cheap from a nutritional viewpoint, and the fine flavor will make it worth every penny. All eggs called for should be from *inoculated immunized chickens*. If not available, use Jolly Joan Egg Replacer. Use the whole egg unless otherwise noted.

In baking whole wheat bread it is important to use as much liquid as possible. The finer the wheat is ground, the more liquid is necessary. Remember, the softer the dough, the lighter the loaf. Too much yeast and too rapid a rising will make a less flavorful bread; yeast enzymes need time to work. (Bread can be made without yeast, but it requires at least 24 hours for rising.) Butter should not be used in bread as a shortening—it inhibits the yeast, with the result that you can never predict what will happen. Sesame oil or olive oil is preferable.

These bread recipes are for both diets, except where contraindicated.

Breads, Muffins, and Pancakes

BASIC YEAST BREAD*

2½ **cups water (or potato water)**
¼ **cup honey**
3 **tablespoons sesame oil**

*Reprinted with permission from A *Mini Guide to Living Foods*, Price-Pottenger Nutrition Foundation, Inc.

1½ teaspoon salt
1½ teaspoon kelp
6 cups freshly ground whole wheat flour
1 tablespoon yeast granules
2 tablespoons water or more
Sesame oil

Mix water, honey, oil, salt, and kelp. Stir well and mix in flour. Cover with a towel and let stand overnight at room temperature. Next morning dissolve yeast granules in 2 or more tablespoons water and work into dough on oiled surface for kneading with oiled hands for 10 minutes. Do not add more flour. Return to oiled bowl, cover, and let rise until double in bulk, one hour at 80° to 85° F. Knead about 2 minutes more and divide into loaves and shape. Grease bread pans and place loaves in them. Let rise another 20 minutes then bake 1 hour and 15 minutes at 325° F. Makes 2 to 3 loaves.

WHOLE WHEAT BREAD

In order to break down the phytic acid in the wheat, it is imperative to allow the freshly ground flour to soak at least 7 hours before baking.

2 packages yeast
2 teaspoons sea salt
⅓ cup oil or softened butter *or* ½ cup applesauce or chopped apples
⅓ cup honey
1 cup rice, freshly ground
2 cups warm water
7 cups whole wheat flour, freshly ground

Ingredients should be at room temperature.

Place first 7 ingredients and 3 cups of the flour in a large mixing bowl.

Beat 8 to 10 minutes with an electric mixer. This helps

develop the gluten protein in the wheat that forms the structure of the bread.

Stir in another 2 cups of flour. It does not need to be smooth.

Sprinkle 1 cup flour in a circle on the kneading surface, and turn out the dough onto this flour.

Oil your hands and knead the flour, using fingertips, only until the dough stiffens up and isn't so sticky.

Continue kneading for 5 to 10 minutes or until dough is smooth and elastic.

Cover with plastic wrap and folded towel; allow to set 20 minutes or so.

Punch down and let rise overnight or 7 hours. If you choose to wait 7 hours, after 6½ place the dough on an oiled surface, and with an oiled rolling pin, divide in two. Roll up toward you, jellyroll fashion, from the small end, sealing well.

Place seam side down in greased bread pans, and brush with oil. Cover with plastic wrap and refrigerate anywhere from 7 to 24 hours.

About 15 minutes before baking, preheat the oven to 375° F and remove dough from the refrigerator. Uncover it, puncture with an oiled toothpick any air bubbles that may have developed, and bake for 30 to 35 minutes. The loaves may be brushed with oil when removed from the oven.

BARLEY BREAD

> **1 cup plus 1 tablespoon barley flour, freshly ground**
> **3 teaspoons Cellu baking powder**
> **¼ teaspoon sea salt**
> **2 teaspoons olive oil**
> **1 tablespoon honey**
> **½ cup water**

Sift the flour before measuring it, and then mix all the dry ingredients. Combine with the oil. Mix the honey and water and add to the dry ingredients. Bake at 300° F for 25 minutes in a small loaf pan that has been oiled.

APRICOT OR PRUNE BREAD

1 cup dried apricots or pitted prunes
¼ cup butter
1 cup frozen orange juice concentrate (undiluted)
2 cups flour, freshly ground
3 heaping teaspoons potassium baking powder
2 tablespoons de-cyanided apricot meal
½ cup chopped nuts

Soak the dried fruit and dice with scissors (or run through a meat grinder). This should yield over 1 cup. Set aside. Place the butter and orange juice in the blender and blend well. Pour this mixture into a mixing bowl. Sift together the flour and baking powder, adding the mixture to the orange juice blend. Add the dried fruit at this point, mixing all together. Finally, add the chopped nuts and the apricot meal. Oil a bread pan and place a piece of brown paper bag, cut to fit, inside the pan. Oil the paper and place the batter on top. Push the batter solidly into the corners of the bread pan and bake at 300° F for 1 hour.

NUT BREAD

1 cup warm potato water
1 package dry yeast
2 tablespoons honey
1 cup corn flour

Blend together and let rise until very light—probably around 45 minutes. Add the following to make a stiff loaf:

½ cup sunflower seed meal, freshly ground
1 cup chopped nuts
1 cup currants
1 teaspoon Jolly Joan Egg Replacer
1 tablespoon olive oil
1 cup ground pumpkin seeds
1 cup bran
1 teaspoon kelp

Don't bother to knead this bread because there is no gluten in it. Stir it with a big spoon, then put it in an oiled bread pan. Let it rise while the oven heats; bake 10 minutes at 400° F and an additional 50 minutes at 350°.

SUNFLOWER SEED CRACKERS

Sunflower seeds in desired amount, finely ground
Water

Mix enough water into the seeds to be able to easily handle. Form into ¼-inch thick patties. Bake in an ungreased glass baking dish until brown. Turn over and brown other side. Serve with a raw marmalade or raw fruit butter, if desired.

PUMPKIN SEED CRACKERS

3 cups freshly ground pumpkin seeds
1 cup freshly ground sesame seeds
¾ teaspoon sea salt
3 tablespoons olive oil
Boiling water

Mix the pumpkin seeds with sesame seeds, salt, and olive oil. Add enough water to make a stiff dough. Oil a cookie sheet, and roll out the dough as thin as possible on the sheet. Dampening your roller will prevent sticking. Cut the dough into desired shape. Bake 30 minutes at 300° F.

Suggestion: Cornmeal or sunflower seeds can be used in place of pumpkin seeds.

CORNMEAL CAKES

2 cups stone ground corn meal
1 teaspoon sesame salt
Boiling water
Olive oil for griddle

Combine meal, salt, and enough liquid to make a thick batter. Drop by tablespoonsful onto a hot, oiled griddle and bake until brown. Serve with butter.

CORNMEAL-RICE MUFFINS

1 cup cooked brown rice
1 cup water
1¼ cups cornmeal (not degerminated)
½ teaspoon salt
2 tablespoons soy flour
¼ cup oil

Mash rice with fork. Bring water to boil in pan that is large enough for mixing muffins. Mix cornmeal, flour, and salt and add all at once to boiling water. Remove at once from fire and stir until moisture is absorbed. Add mashed rice and mix well with fork. Add oil. Beat. Fill greased muffin pans (make the finished muffins as large as you want and round nicely; they will not rise any higher), or place in mounds on greased cookie sheet. Bake at 300° F for 30 minutes or until nicely browned. Yield 8 muffins.

APPLE-OATMEAL MUFFINS

1 cup shredded raw apple
1½ cups rolled oats
¼ cup oil
½ teaspoon salt
½ cup raisins or chopped dates
¼ cup chopped nuts

Wash apples, quarter, and core. Shred cut-side down on medium shredder. Combine with other ingredients. Let stand for a few minutes to absorb moisture then mix well. Spoon into greased muffin pans. Bake at 300° F for 30 minutes or until browned. Makes 1 to 2 dozen.

BUCKWHEAT PANCAKES

1 cup organic buckwheat flour, freshly ground
1 teaspoon sea salt
1¼ cups water
Olive oil for griddle

Combine ingredients (except oil) and stir well, beating with a hand or electric beater until bubbly. Fry on a griddle that is greased well with olive oil. Serve with raw fruit marmalade if you wish.

SOURDOUGH BUCKWHEAT PANCAKES

½ cup warm water
1 tablespoon raw honey
1 teaspoon El Molino Dry Yeast
1 tablespoon butter, melted
½ teaspoon kelp or sea salt
1½ cups water
1½ cups buckwheat flour, freshly ground in mini mill
1½ cups wheat berries, freshly ground

Stir the honey into ½ cup water until dissolved, and add the yeast. Stir until well mixed and let stand 5 minutes. Add the remaining ingredients to the yeast mixture and beat together. Cover with a towel, and let stand overnight to develop the sour-dough flavor. Drop by spoonsful onto a griddle and bake on both sides. These cakes can be served with raw applesauce.

CASHEW-OAT WAFFLES

2¼ cups water
1½ cups rolled oats
⅓ cup raw cashew nuts
1 tablespoon oil
½ teaspoon salt

Combine all ingredients and blend (in blender) until light and foamy, about half a minute. Let stand while waffle iron is heating. The batter thickens on standing. Blend again briefly. Bake in hot waffle iron 8 to 10 minutes or until nicely browned. Set timer for 8 minutes and do not open before time is up. If iron is hard to open, leave a few seconds longer.

SOUPS

Take any combination of the recommended raw vegetables, page 159, with tomatoes, potatoes, and carrots in particular, and cut in small pieces or liquefy in a blender to shorten cooking time. Raw vegetables can also be covered with water and cooked at a low heat. Cook only enough for one day. Barley, brown rice, or millet may be added. Season with herbs, garlic, or kelp.

RAW AVOCADO TOMATO SOUP

5 large, ripe tomatoes, chopped
1 ripe avocado, sliced
1 green onion, chopped
¼ teaspoon ground dill seed
A dash of cayenne pepper
¼ cup ground almonds
1 cup broth or water
1 teaspoon kelp
Seasoned salt to taste (optional)

Blend all the ingredients with four of the tomatoes. Heat below 115° F just to warm the soup. Chop the last tomato into the soup and serve.

CREAM OF CARROT SOUP

  2 cups Almond Milk, page 164
  1 cup diced raw carrots
  1 small onion, chopped
  2 tablespoons butter
  1 teaspoon kelp
  Herb seasoned salt, to taste
  2 teaspoons vegetable broth seasoning, or to taste

Blend all ingredients, warm and serve.

  Note: There are many variations of seasoning. Experiment and create your very own taste.

CREAM OF PARSNIP SOUP

  1½ parsnips, cubed
  2 cups water

Blend for a few minutes until well pureed. Add:

  ½ medium onion, chopped
  2 to 3 teaspoons olive oil
  1½ cups corn
  1 cup water
  Salt, to taste

Warm to 115° F and serve.

RAW GREEN SOUP

  1 to 2 cups hot water
  2 tablespoons Dr. Jensen's Broth Seasoning
  1 teaspoon kelp
  ½ cup chopped parsley
  ½ cup chopped celery, with tops
  ½ cup chopped spinach leaves
  ½ cup chopped mild-tasting leaf lettuce or watercress
    (if available)
  Butter (optional)

Blend all ingredients with 1 cup of hot water, adding the remaining cup if you see the need. Serve warmed with a pat of butter.

RAW ASPARAGUS SOUP

2 cups hot water
¼ cup ground almonds (use mini mill)
2 cups raw asparagus or 1 package frozen chopped
1 small celery stalk, with tops, chopped
1 small bunch parsley, chopped
A dash of oregano
A pinch of thyme
1 teaspoon herb seasoned salt

Blend together the almonds and hot water for 2 minutes. Add the remaining ingredients and blend until smooth. Serve warmed.

HOMEMADE VEGETABLE BROTH

1 quart saved vegetable trimmings
2 cloves garlic
1 onion, chopped
1 tablespoon herb seasoned salt
1 tablespoon lemon juice or cider vinegar
Water

Place all the ingredients in a pot with enough water to cover the mixture. Cover and simmer for about one hour. Cool the mixture and strain it. Discard vegetables. Keep it refrigerated in a glass jar.

Suggestions: Use this broth for gravies, drinks, soups, or any other such recipes.

POTATO SOUP

1 quart diced potatoes *or* Jerusalem artichokes
3 onions, chopped

1 tablespoon vegetable broth seasoning or salt, to taste
2 quarts water
4 tablespoons butter

Combine vegetables, seasoning, and water. Simmer until all the vegetables are soft. Add butter and serve. Makes 6 cups.

MINESTRONE SOUP

1½ cups mixed beans (kidney, black,
    pinto, navy, red, or split peas)
1 quart water
1 large clove garlic, minced
2 large tomatoes, chopped
2 tablespoons olive oil
1 large onion, sliced coarsely
3 stalks celery, sliced thin
2 medium carrots, chopped
1 bunch chard or spinach, chopped
2 teaspoons sea salt or tamari (optional)

Add the beans to the water and bring to a boil. Cover and boil an additional ten minutes. Let sit covered for one hour. Return to heat and cook with the garlic until beans are tender. Sauté the onion, celery, carrots, tomatoes, and greens. Add to the cooked beans. Allow to cook uncovered 15 or more minutes. Add seasoning and serve. Makes 6 cups.

BORSCHT

4 cups water
4 to 5 beets, grated
4 tablespoons tamari
1 cup chopped beet greens
1 teaspoon dill weed
1 green onion, chopped

Bring the water with beets and tamari to a boil. Cover and simmer 10 minutes. Add the remaining ingredients and simmer for 10 minutes more. Serve warm, cold, or room temperature.

STEAMED GREEN SOUP

> 1 cup steamed chard or spinach
> 3 cups hot Homemade Vegetable Broth, page 183
> 1 tablespoon arrowroot
> 1 tablespoon butter
> ¼ cup mushrooms, finely sliced
> Cream (optional)

Blend first 3 ingredients until soup thickens. Add butter and mushrooms. Cream may be added if you so desire.

BLACK BEAN SOUP

> 4 cups water
> 1 cup black beans
> 2 tablespoons olive oil
> 2 onions, sliced
> 1 stalk celery, sliced
> ½ teaspoon herb seasoned salt
> 1 bay leaf
> ¼ teaspoon celery seed
> ¼ teaspoon basil
> Juice of 1 lemon
> 1 cup vegetable broth
> Season salt, to taste

Cook the beans in 4 cups water for ten minutes. Let sit one hour. Simmer with one onion until tender. Sauté the other onion and celery in the olive oil. Set aside. Puree the bean soup in your blender, and add the remaining ingredients. Simmer 15 minutes or more. Season and serve. Makes 3 cups.

WHOLE GRAIN SOUP

1 clove garlic, minced
2 onions, chopped
1 stalk celery, sliced thinly
1 tablespoon olive oil
1 cup brown rice (or millet, rye, wheat berries, barley, or oat groats)
4 cups boiling water
¼ lb. mushrooms, sliced
2 tablespoons tamari
1 teaspoon kelp

Gently warm the garlic, onion, and celery in the oil. Add your choice of grain and lightly sauté with the vegetables until golden. Add boiling water and simmer 1 hour or more. Gently warm the mushrooms by adding them to the soup once it is removed from the heat. Add the tamari and kelp.

VEGETABLE SOUP

4 carrots
2 onions
4 stalks celery
½ lb. green beans
Garlic, minced
½ cup water (or more if needed)
2 to 4 cups of tomatoes, blended
1 small beet, grated
⅛ cup butter
½ cabbage, shredded
2 tablespoons Dr. Jensen's Broth Seasoning, or to taste
1 teaspoon kelp

Chop the first five ingredients listed. Add to water and steam for approximately 10 minutes. Add blended tomatoes, beets, butter, and cabbage; simmer 3 minutes longer. Serve.

MISO

  ½ cup dry dulse or wakame (seaweed)
  1 cup water
  Olive oil
  1 large onion, sliced
  1 cup cabbage, shredded coarsely
  1 carrot, sliced
  Spinach, chopped
  2 cups water
  1 tablespoon miso paste, or to taste

Soak the seaweed for 15 minutes in 1 cup of water and then cut into pieces. Sauté the onion, cabbage, carrot, and spinach in oil for 5 minutes. Add remaining 2 cups of water and the wakame. Simmer 20 minutes more. Dilute the miso in a cup with a small amount of the above broth and add to the soup. Stir well and serve. Makes 3 cups.

CREAM OF VEGETABLE SOUP

  Butter
  ½ cup corn, fresh or frozen
  ½ cup peas, fresh or frozen
  ½ cup limas, fresh or frozen
  Several raw mushrooms, sliced
  ½ red or green bell pepper
  1 small garlic clove, pressed
  1 green onion, coarsely chopped
  2 cups Almond Milk (see page 164)
  1 teaspoon kelp
  Vegetable broth seasoning, to taste
  Herb seasoned salt, to taste

Warm in melted butter the corn, peas, limas and mushrooms. Let sit covered for a few minutes. Blend all the remaining ingredients together and add to the warmed vegetables. Serve warm.

LENTIL SOUP

1½ cups lentils
4 cups water
1 onion, chopped
1 teaspoon herb seasoned salt
1 teaspoon kelp
1 large garlic clove, pressed
1 carrot, grated
2 tomatoes, chopped

Simmer all ingredients except the carrots and tomatoes for 1 to 2 hours. Add the grated carrot and chopped tomatoes before serving.

RAW VEGETABLE SOUP

Butter
½ cup chopped celery
2 tomatoes, cut in small pieces
1 onion, chopped
2 parsley sprigs, chopped
½ cup finely shredded cabbage
Spinach leaves, chopped fine
1 quart water
1 cup grated carrots
1 cup fresh peas
1 beet, grated
A dash of garlic powder
Vegetable broth seasoning, to taste

Melt the butter, and gently warm the celery, tomatoes, onion, parsley, cabbage and spinach leaves in it. Do not cook. Place the lid on your pan and let it sit for a few minutes. Meanwhile, heat water to under 130° F. Add the warmed vegetables, garlic powder, and seasoning. Place blended mixture back in the pan with the remaining ingredients, and warm them all together— lightly.

CREAM OF MUSHROOM SOUP
(For Non-Strict Diet)

½ lb. mushrooms, sliced (a larger amount may be used)
Soy milk
1 oz. sunflower seeds
1 small garlic clove, pressed
1 small onion, chopped
1 small celery stalk with leaves, chopped

Warm all the ingredients together (130° F) and then blend. Add a few more sliced raw mushrooms before serving.

Suggestion: This soup can be made with Almond Milk (¼ cup almonds blended two minutes with one cup of water) instead of soy milk.

SALADS

Vegetables high in abscisins, such as onions, carrots, beets, turnips, kohlrabi, celery root, Jerusalem artichokes, potatoes, radishes, and parsnips should be used with cabbage, chard, endive, lettuce, parsley, and spinach. Tomatoes, broccoli, cauliflower, peas, peppers, and corn are good choices, as are lightly steamed lima beans, snap beans, eggplant, and pumpkins. Raw vegetables offer unlimited combinations to be used according to personal preference.

When preparing salads, remember that grating, chopping, and slicing expose the vegetables to oxygen and oxidation. Once exposed, vegetables should be consumed immediately, as they will deteriorate rapidly. So make your salad just before you are ready to eat it so you don't lose all the precious nutrients.

Use only the salad dressing recipes given in this book. *Do not* purchase ready-made salad dressings as they are often full of chemicals and preservatives or made with poor oils.

Note: Carefully wash and peel all fruits and vegetables that are not organically grown.

GREEN GARDEN SALAD

2 cups garbanzo beans, cooked
½ cup sunflower seeds
2 tomatoes, sliced
4 romaine lettuce leaves, shredded
Small handful raw pumpkin seeds
1 carrot, sliced thin
Flowers from 2 broccoli stalks
2 broccoli stalks, chopped

Combine the ingredients, tossing lightly, saving the sliced broccoli and flowers for a topping decoration. Serve with Green Goddess Dressing, page 200. Serves 4.

BEET SALAD

Shredded raw beets
Chopped onion

Marinate beets and onions together in homemade French Dressing, pages 197 and 198. Serve on chopped salad greens.

CABBAGE-CARROT SALAD

1 quarter head cabbage
1 carrot
1 Jerusalem artichoke, chopped
1 small apple, chopped
Eggless Mayonnaise with sesame salt (see page 199)
Papaya seed pepper

Grate the carrot and cabbage into a bowl. Add artichoke and apple. Use just enough mayonnaise to moisten. Add papaya seed pepper.

CABBAGE-PINEAPPLE SALAD

2 cups shredded cabbage
¼ cup chopped fresh pineapple
1 apple, chopped
⅓ cup homemade dressing
Sprinkle of seasoned kelp (SeaZun)
1/16 teaspoon ground papaya seed pepper
Herb seasoned salt, to taste

Mix well and serve. The cabbage core has many nutrients. Try eating some while preparing your salad.

ARTICHOKE SALAD

6 Jerusalem artichokes, grated
2 carrots, grated
3 stalks celery, chopped fine
1 apple, chopped fine
¾ cup finely shredded cabbage
¼ cup chopped parsley
A few pumpkin seeds

Mix and serve with Eggless Mayonnaise (see page 199) that has kelp and red cayenne pepper added to it.

BEET 'N APPLE SALAD

2 medium beets, grated fine
1 apple, chopped well
1 tablespoon almond butter
1 tablespoon lemon juice
2 tablespoons water

Mix the grated beets and chopped apple together in a bowl. Mix together the almond butter, lemon juice and water, and pour over your salad.

CARROT, CELERY, APPLE SALAD

1 celery stalk, chopped fine
2 carrots, grated
1 apple, diced
A dash of cinnamon
½ cup cashews
¼ cup apple juice

Mix together first three ingredients in a bowl. Blend together the cashews, juice, and cinnamon. Serve as a dressing over the salad.

ASPARAGUS MUSHROOM SALAD

Several raw mushrooms, sliced
½ cup finely sliced young asparagus tips, raw
⅛ cup finely chopped chives
¼ cup cubed Jerusalem artichoke
½ cup coarsely chopped walnuts

Mix ingredients together and serve with kelp, cayenne, seasoned Eggless Mayonnaise *or* Lemon and Oil Dressing, pages 199 and 200.

GOLDEN GLOW SUPREME

Carrots, grated
1 beet, grated
Zucchini, grated
Red pepper, finely chopped
Green onions, finely chopped
Red apples, diced fine
Pumpkin seeds, raw
Eggless Mayonnaise I or II, page 199
A few tablespoons pineapple juice
Lettuce or greens
Pineapple, cubed

Mix together in a bowl the first seven ingredients. Prepare a simple dressing from the mayonnaise and pineapple juice. Dress the salad and place in a mound on top of the greens. Surround it with pineapple chunks.

GOLDEN BEET SALAD

1 teaspoon arrowroot
¼ cup beet juice
¾ cup orange juice
⅛ cup lemon juice
1 tablespoon apple cider vinegar
1½ tablespoons honey
½ teaspoon sea salt
1 heaping teaspoon ascorbic acid crystals
4 cups sliced beets, steamed
1 tablespoon orange rind, grated
2 tablespoons butter

Mix the arrowroot with the beet juice, and stir until smooth. Add the orange juice, lemon juice, vinegar, honey and sea salt. Cook until clear and thickened. When cooled a bit add ascorbic acid. Add the beets, orange rind, and butter. Serve warm.

MARINATED ZUCCHINI MUSHROOM SALAD

1 zucchini, grated
2 green onions, chopped
Several large mushrooms, sliced
½ bunch parsley, chopped fine
1 tomato, sliced
A sprinkle of sunflower seeds
1 Jerusalem artichoke, sliced thin

Toss all the ingredients with Herb Tomato Dressing, page 198, and serve.

CAULIFLOWER CARROT PECAN SALAD

1½ cups chopped cauliflower buds
1 cup coarsely grated carrots
¾ cup chopped green pepper
1 cup chopped celery
1 cup pecan halves

Mix together and dress with Horseradish Mayonnaise, page 197.
Serve on green leaves. Serves 4 to 6.

MUSHROOM MARINADE

½ lb. mushrooms, sliced
¼ teaspoon herb seasoned salt
½ teaspoon oregano
1 tablespoon lemon juice
½ cup olive oil (pure)

Mix the marinade ingredients with the mushrooms and let stand
2 to 3 hours at room temperature or overnight if more convenient.

STUFFED AVOCADOS

Red pepper, chopped
Onion, chopped
Cucumber, chopped
Mushrooms *or* cauliflower buds, chopped small
Tomato, cut into small pieces
Eggless Mayonnaise, page 199
Kelp
Cayenne pepper
Avocados

Toss all the vegetables (finely chopped) with mayonnaise that has
been seasoned with kelp and cayenne. Serve in avocado halves
on a lettuce leaf.

CABBAGE GLOW SALAD

Romaine lettuce or other leaf lettuce
½ cup chopped or finely shredded purple cabbage
1 carrot, grated
1 beet, grated
1 stalk celery, finely chopped

Place the lettuce leaves on a plate with the cabbage in the center, carrots and beets mixed with celery surrounding them. Dress with Horseradish Mayonnaise, page 197, or with the dressing of your choice.

GARDEN SALAD SUPREME

Green leafy vegetable of your choice
Grated or chopped:

Cucumbers	**Turnips**
Green onions	**Jerusalem artichokes**
Beets	**Tomatoes**
Parsley	**Avocado wedges**
Pumpkin seeds	
1 teaspoon kelp	

Mix all ingredients, using the tomatoes and avocado wedges on top. Serve with your favorite dressing.

ARTICHOKE SALAD

1 cup grated Jerusalem artichokes
½ cup grated beets
1 avocado, sliced into wedges
Lettuce

Mix together the beets and artichokes, placing on a lettuce bed. Place the avocado wedges around, and dress with Lemon and Oil Dressing, page 201.

RAW POTATO SALAD

Juice of ¼ lemon
2 cups grated potatoes (medium size)
Water
1 stalk celery, chopped
1 green onion, chopped
1 teaspoon ascorbic acid crystals
1 teaspoon celery seeds
1 cup diced cucumbers
1 teaspoon dill seeds
1 teaspoon kelp or sea salt, to taste
Eggless Mayonnaise, page 199

Add the lemon juice to the grated potatoes and enough water to cover. Let soak for 5 minutes. Drain (the liquid may be added to juice). Add the remaining ingredients and mayonnaise to taste, and garnish with paprika and parsley. —

VEGETABLE MOLD I

1 tablespoon vegetable gelatin
¼ cup water
1¾ cup water *or* tomato juice
1 to 2 tablespoons Dr. Jensen's Broth Seasoning, to taste
1 tablespoon lemon juice
1 heaping teaspoon ascorbic acid crystals
A dash of cayenne pepper
1½ cups any combination of chopped vegetables
    (e.g., onions, peppers, celery, cabbage, and carrots)

Melt the gelatin and the water over low heat. Mix together in blender the water (or juice) with the broth seasoning, lemon juice, ascorbic acid crystals, and cayenne. Add the gelatin while this is blending. Place in a mold or bowl and refrigerate until the consistency of egg white. Add the vegetables at this time. Let firm. Serve with homemade dressing.

Salad Dressings

HORSERADISH DRESSING

¼ cup olive oil
4 teaspoons lemon juice
⅓ teaspoon Dijon-type French mustard
1 clove of garlic, crushed
1 teaspoon fresh horseradish
⅛ teaspoon ground papaya seed pepper
¼ teaspoon seasoning salt to taste

Mix all ingredients in blender. Serve over tomatoes and cucumbers.

POPPY SEED DRESSING

¼ cup poppy seed
¼ cup unsweetened pineapple juice (fresh or frozen)
1 medium onion
1 teaspoon kelp
Sea salt, to taste
¼ teaspoon paprika
2 teaspoons lemon juice
2 teaspoons honey
¼ cup olive oil

Blend together all ingredients except the oil. Turning blender on a low speed, add the oil very slowly. Add a few more seeds and stir in. Chill until ready to serve. Makes 2 cups.

FRENCH DRESSING

3 tablespoons olive oil
1 tablespoon lemon juice
1 teaspoon powdered mustard (optional)

½ teaspoon herbed seasoning
¼ teaspoon kelp
1 crushed garlic clove
¼ teaspoon papaya seed pepper (Save seeds from papaya, wash and dry well, and grind in pepper mill. Adds zest to dishes and aids digestion.)

Blend well. Use as desired.

TOASTED SESAME DRESSING

¼ cup ground sesame seeds, toasted dry in a skillet until lightly browned
⅔ cup water
¼ teaspoon kelp
¼ teaspoon papaya seed pepper
Juice of ½ lemon
Herb seasoned salt, if desired

Blend all ingredients together well. Makes ½ cup.

HERB TOMATO DRESSING

2 tomatoes
1 clove garlic
¼ cup lemon juice, or to taste
¼ cup olive oil
1 teaspoon kelp
1 or more teaspoons Dr. Jensen's Broth Seasoning
¼ teaspoon each:
basil,
oregano,
thyme,
marjoram

Blend together everything except the oil; add that slowly to the blending mixture in a fine stream.

GUACAMOLE

2 medium avocados
Juice of ½ lemon
¼ cup Eggless Mayonnaise, page 199
1 small clove garlic
1 small onion, sliced
½ teaspoon cayenne pepper
Herbed salt, to taste

Blend all ingredients in blender and chill.

Suggestion: Thin with more mayonnaise or whipping cream and use as a salad dressing.

EGGLESS MAYONNAISE I

½ cup cashews
1 teaspoon kelp
1 teaspoon SeaZun
1 teaspoon Herba Mare
½ teaspoon paprika (omit for Strict Diet.)

Pulverize in blender. Now add slowly to blender:

1 cup water
1 clove garlic
½ cup oil
1 tablespoon cider vinegar *or* lemon juice

Makes 1 pint.

EGGLESS MAYONNAISE II

¼ cup lemon juice *or* apple cider vinegar
1 teaspoon honey
2 tablespoons tahini
¼ teaspoon Herba Mare
⅛ teaspoon SeaZun
¼ cup olive oil

Mix the first five ingredients in blender. Add olive oil very slowly—as much as needed to thicken to your preference. Store in glass jar in refrigerator. Makes 1 cup.

CUCUMBER DRESSING

1 tablespoon chopped green onion
½ cucumber peeled and chopped
Juice of lemon
¼ cup olive oil
¼ teaspoon herb seasoned salt
¼ teaspoon paprika
1 teaspoon tamari

Blend all ingredients until smooth and adjust seasoning to taste.

CREAM OF TOMATO DRESSING

3 tomatoes
1 tablespoon lemon juice (or to taste)
1 tablespoon or more sesame butter
Herb seasoned salt, to taste and/or garlic powder to taste

Blend well. Makes 1 cup of dressing.

GREEN GODDESS DRESSING

½ cup Eggless Mayonnaise, page 199
¾ cup chopped parsley
1 teaspoon chopped onion
1 small piece garlic, sliced
Herb seasoned salt (optional)
½ teaspoon kelp
1 tablespoon water or more

Blend all ingredients in a blender. Add more water if needed.

LEMON AND OIL DRESSING

1 to 2 teaspoons honey, raw
1 tablespoon lemon juice
¼ teaspoon kelp
A dash cayenne (optional)
½ cup olive oil
Herb seasoned salt, to taste

Combine the ingredients well. Makes ¾ cup.

VEGETABLES AND LEGUMES

Use only fresh, naturally grown vegetables that have not been sprayed with pesticides or chemicals. Canned and frozen vegetables are lacking in nutrients, especially the vitamin A analogs, which are easily destroyed by processing. We choose many root vegetables and seeds, and we include the stems and ends of stems of mature greens as well as the leaves.

Broccoli and cauliflower are excellent vegetables for your diet, because their flowering heads are preparing to set seeds. (If you grow your own vegetables, the flowering parts of the vegetables are good sources of the nutrients you need. The blossoms of broccoli, cauliflower, and squash will be a colorful as well as a nutritive addition to your salads.)

Choose large, well-formed vegetables past the stage of rapid growth: those about to go to seed or set fruit, and those about to go dormant, which are storing their energy in their roots or tubers.

Carefully wash all vegetables to remove any contaminants. Scrub your root vegetables and potatoes well, but do not remove the skins. Much of the mineral content is contained in or near the skin, and if the vegetables are naturally grown you will want to utilize all of it.

Think in terms of eating the whole vegetable. For example, abscisins are present in the stems where the plant joins at the base (e.g., the wide end of the celery and the bottom ends of beets). Don't throw away the parts that contain the valuable abscisins your body needs now.

Vegetables should be cooked in waterless cookware or steamed in a steamer with a little water at low heat. Conserve all juices. You can either drink them as they are or add them to soups or other juices. Vegetables may be served with a salt-free dressing or herb or kelp seasoning.

Vegetable Dishes

SWEET POTATOES

Preheat oven to 300° F. Scrub the sweet potatoes thoroughly and pat dry. Bake for 45 minutes to one hour until soft to the touch. Serve with raw butter, if desired, and some sesame salt or herb seasoned salt.

Suggestions: Potatoes may also be steamed in a stainless steel steaming basket, in waterless cookware with a small amount of water, or in a pottery steaming crock for 30 to 45 minutes or until desired softness is reached. Serve sweet potatoes 3 times a week.

STEAMED TURNIPS

3 medium turnips, cut in slices or pieces
Water to cover bottom of pan
Raw butter

Use a collapsible steamer basket (which allows vegetables to cook quickly with a minimum of attention), vapor cook, or use a ceramic steamer. Bring water to a boil. Lower heat and lightly steam. Add raw butter to taste.

BAKED WHITE POTATOES

White potatoes
Oil
Raw butter (optional)
Sesame salt *or* herb seasoned salt

Preheat oven to 300° F. Scrub white potatoes thoroughly and pat dry. Rub them with oil and bake 45 minutes to one hour, until soft to the touch. Serve with raw butter if desired and some sesame salt or herb seasoned salt.

Suggestions: Potatoes may also be steamed in waterless cookware with a small amount of water in a stainless steel steaming basket, or in a pottery steaming crock for 30 to 45 minutes, or until desired softness is obtained.

SIMPLY EGGPLANT

Eggplant
Butter

Slice eggplant rather thinly and dot with butter. Broil on a cookie sheet just until tender. It is not necessary to turn it.

Suggestion: If there are other foods you are broiling, place the eggplant under the rack on which these foods will be placed. The eggplant will baste in these drippings.

ASPARAGUS
WITH MUSHROOM SAUCE

2 medium bunches of asparagus
Water, if steaming
Raw Mushroom Sauce, page 223

Snap off the bottom 2 to 3 inches of tough stalk, and slice the rest into bite size pieces. Use raw or steam lightly. Place on a lettuce bed and pour the mushroom sauce on top.

SPICY CARROTS

> 3 cups sliced carrots
> 1 cup apple juice
> ½ teaspoon sea salt
> 1 tablespoon raw butter
> 1½ teaspoons grated orange peel
> 1½ teaspoons grated lemon peel

Cover the carrots with the apple juice and simmer in a covered pot until tender. Water may be added if necessary. Continue simmering until the liquid becomes syrupy. Add the remaining ingredients and serve.

GRATED SQUASH

> ¼ stick butter
> 3 cups grated squash or pumpkin
> ½ teaspoon seasame salt
> A dash of cinnamon or nutmeg (optional)

Warm the butter, adding all the ingredients. Warm and toss this mixture for 15 minutes. Serves 4.

Main Dishes

CARROT PEA PATTIES

> 2 cups fresh peas
> 2 cups grated raw carrots
> 1 green onion, chopped
> 1 red pepper, chopped
> ½ cup ground sunflower seeds
> A dash of cayenne
> 2 teaspoons kelp, herbs and seasoning to taste

Grind all ingredients together with a meat grinder. Form into patties and serve with Eggless Mayonnaise, page 199.

CAULIFLOWER WITH HERB CREAM SAUCE

1 cup Almond *or* Cashew Milk, pages 164 and 165
¼ teaspoon sea salt
½ teaspoon kelp
¼ teaspoon tarragon, sweet basil, and savory
Vegetable broth powder, if desired
1 head cauliflower, sliced fine
Water, if steaming is desired
1 tablespoon butter

Mix together the nut milk and all the seasoning and herbs. Warm the mixture by steaming slightly or prepare raw. Toss in the finely sliced cauliflower, and serve on a lettuce bed. Sprinkle the top with paprika.

RAW SUCCOTASH

2 cups fresh corn
2 cups fresh lima beans
2 green onions, finely chopped
2 celery stalks, chopped
1 tomato, chopped
A small amount of cayenne pepper
1 tablespoon Dr. Jensen's Broth Seasoning
1 teaspoon kelp

Mix all ingredients and warm gently, then serve.

HERBED MILLET

1 cup millet
3 cups vegetable broth or water
Red cayenne pepper, to taste
½ teaspoon kelp, or as desired
½ bunch parsley, chopped fine
1 teaspoon herb seasoned salt
Butter
½ cup slivered nuts (optional)

Boil water or broth and then add the millet. Cover and simmer for 15 to 20 minutes, or longer if needed. The millet should be light and fluffy. *Do not stir* during the cooking time. Add the remaining ingredients and adjust seasoning. Makes 3 cups.

SPANISH RICE

1 tablespoon butter
3 tablespoons chopped celery
3 tablespoons chopped onion
3 tablespoons chopped green pepper
¼ cup Homemade Tomato Sauce, page 224
Cayenne pepper, to taste
1 clove garlic, pressed
2 cups cooked brown rice
Sea salt, to taste
½ cup sliced almonds (optional)

Gently melt the butter. Warm, don't cook, the celery, onion, and green pepper in it, tossing until lightly golden. Warm the tomato sauce, adding the cayenne and garlic, in a separate pan. Combine all the ingredients with the rice, adding salt.

BUCKWHEAT GROAT VEGETABLE STUFFING

⅛ cup butter
1 large onion, chopped
½ cup chopped celery
½ cup green pepper, chopped
½ cup chopped zucchini, or more if desired
1 teaspoon kelp
1 cup buckwheat groats
1 to 2 teaspoons sesame salt
2 cups boiling water
Desired herbs
½ cup cashews (optional)

Melt butter in the pan, and add the vegetables. Heat until yellowed and barely softened. Add the remaining ingredients; cover and steam about 20 minutes, then serve.

TABOULI

> 1 cup warm water
> 2 cups bulgur wheat
> 1 cup chopped parsley
> ½ cup chopped onion
> 2 tomatoes, chopped
> 2 tablespoons fresh mint *or* 1 tablespoon dried
> 1 cup lemon juice
> ¼ cup olive oil
> Papaya seed pepper
> Sea salt, to taste
> ½ cup pine nuts (optional)

Soak the wheat in warm water 1 hour. Add the other ingredients, toss. Refrigerate before serving to allow the wheat to absorb the moisture. Serve on a bed of lettuce.

CURRIED BULGUR

> ⅓ cup bulgur wheat
> ⅔ cup water
> Butter
> 2 stalks celery, chopped
> 1 teaspoon kelp
> 1 small onion, chopped
> ½ teaspoon curry powder
> ⅓ cup chopped walnuts (optional)

Boil the water and add the bulgur. Simmer for 15 minutes. In a separate pan melt the butter, add the vegetables, and gently warm. Mix all the ingredients together and enjoy.

VEGETABLE SEED BURGERS

½ cup grated carrots
½ cup very finely chopped celery
1 green onion, finely chopped
1 tablespoon chopped parsley
1 tablespoon chopped red bell pepper
1 tablespoon olive oil
1 cup ground sunflower seeds
Dr. Jensen's Broth Seasoning, to taste
½ teaspoon kelp
Water
¼ cup chopped hazelnuts (optional)

Combine the ingredients with enough water to hold together the mixture. Form into patties and bake in an oiled baking dish at the lowest possible temperature until dry and somewhat firm. Serves 4.

WILD RICE WITH VEGETABLES

⅔ cup wild rice
3 cups water
2 stalks celery, chopped
1 onion, chopped
1 green pepper, chopped
Butter
Sea salt, if needed
1 tablespoon Dr. Jensen's Broth Seasoning
½ cup pine nuts (optional)

Wash the rice well. Boil the water and pour over the rice; cover and simmer until tender, approximately 45 minutes. Lightly sauté the celery, onion, and green pepper in butter. Add these vegetables and the seasoning to the wild rice. Sprinkle with nuts. Serves 4.

VEGETABLE MEAT BALLS

1½ cups ground sesame seeds
½ cup ground sunflower seeds
1 red pepper, chopped fine
4 green onions, chopped fine
1 tablespoon ground dill seed
¾ to 1 cup water
2 teaspoons Dr. Jensen's Broth Seasoning, or to taste

Mix all ingredients, adding broth or seasoned water last. Add enough water to get a firm consistency, like ground beef. Shape into meat balls and place in the oven at the lowest possible temperature—just long enough to dry the outside. Serve with a tomato sauce or vegetables.

ZUCCHINI ONION DISH IN SAUCE

1 stalk celery, chopped
1 medium zucchini, shredded
½ green pepper, chopped
1 small onion, minced
Sesame salt, to taste (optional)
Melted butter *(do not allow to brown)*
⅛ teaspoon garlic powder
Tofu
Homemade Tomato Sauce, page 224

Mix together in a baking dish the celery, zucchini, onion, and green pepper. Lightly salt if desired. Mix the garlic powder in the butter and dribble over the vegetables. Break up some tofu on top of the vegetables. Warm the tomato sauce lightly (do not cook) and pour over the ingredients. Lightly toss and place it in the oven at the lowest possible temperature. Do not cook. Keep the temperature at or below 110° so that the ingredients just warm together briefly. Serve with ¼ cup nuts per serving.

SPAGHETTI SQUASH

Spaghetti squash
Butter
Herb seasoned salt
Mushroom Spaghetti Sauce, or Homemade Tomato Sauce,
**   pages 214 and 224**

Place the squash in a baking glass with ¼″ water in the bottom.
Puncture the squash with a fork to prevent it from exploding.
Bake at 300° F for 45 minutes to 1 hour. Squash will give slightly
when pressed with your hand. Slice it lengthwise or crosswise
and scoop out the spaghetti with a fork. (Serve seeds with squash
if desired.) Serve this delicious squash in place of pasta for spaghetti or enjoy plain with butter and herbs.

WOK VEGETABLES

1 small stalk broccoli, chopped
2 stalks celery, chopped diagonally
1 onion, sliced
½ cup shredded cabbage
Mushrooms, sliced
2 tablespoons olive oil
¼ teaspoon garlic powder
¼ teaspoon tarragon
¼ teaspoon sweet basil
Sesame salt, to taste
½ cup sliced almonds

In a wok sauté the broccoli, celery, and onions for 10 minutes.
Add the remaining vegetables and sauté 5 minutes more. Season
while cooking and serve.

CURRIED VEGETABLES

2 tablespoons olive oil
2 onions, chopped

½ lb. cauliflower florets
½ lb. broccoli, chopped
Curry powder, to taste
¼ cup almonds, toasted or raw, ground if desired
2 tablespoons currants

Sauté vegetables until tender and add the curry powder. Add the nuts and currants last. Serve over millet or brown rice.

STUFFED ZUCCHINI

2 large zucchini
½ cup finely chopped asparagus tips,
    raw or steamed lightly
¼ cup chopped onion
1 cup finely chopped mushrooms
1 tomato, chopped well
½ teaspoon oregano or sweet basil
2 oz. sesame seeds, ground
⅓ cup water
1 tablespoon Dr. Jensen's Broth Seasoning
1 tablespoon nutritional yeast

Slice the zucchini lengthwise, scooping out the inner meat. Steam the empty shells for 5 minutes. Grate the scooped out zucchini and add the asparagus, onion, mushrooms, tomato, and herbs. Place the ground sesame seeds in the blender with the water, broth seasoning, and yeast. Blend until smooth. Mix this spread with tossed vegetables and stuff inside the steamed zucchini shells. Serve with ¼ cup nuts per person.

STUFFED ACORN SQUASH

2 acorn squash
2 tablespoons olive oil
1 medium onion, chopped fine
1 carrot, grated

1 cup peas
½ cup sliced mushrooms
1 stalk celery, chopped fine
3 tablespoons ground sesame seeds
Sea salt, to taste
⅓ cup pine nuts

Cut the squash in half, clean, and bake with cut side down in a baking dish 40 minutes or longer. A knife inserted easily in skin indicates squash is done. Meanwhile, toss the remaining ingredients and stuff this mixture into the halved squash. Sprinkle nuts on top. Return to the oven and lightly warm. Do not cook the vegetables. Sprinkle with paprika and serve.

CAULIFLOWER WITH HERB CREAM SAUCE

1 cup Almond or Cashew Milk, pages 164 and 165
¼ teaspoon sea salt
½ teaspoon kelp
¼ cup finely chopped parsley
½ teaspoon tarragon, sweet basil, and savory
Vegetable broth powder (optional)
1 head cauliflower, sliced fine, steamed if desired
Water, if steaming
1 tablespoon butter, if steaming
½ cup chopped cashews

Mix together the nut milk with all the seasonings and herbs. Warm the mixture. *Do not cook.* Toss in the sliced raw or steamed cauliflower and serve on a lettuce bed. Sprinkle the top with paprika and chopped cashews.

RICE-AND-CURRY PARTY FOOD

Among the advantages of this meal is the fact that most of the ingredients are served separately, so that a variety of people with various food restrictions can serve themselves from the same buffet line, each avoiding his or her personally incompatable foods. Most of the condiments offered are raw. It is a complete meal in itself without the addition of extra side dishes beyond a raw finger vegetable assortment of perhaps carrot, celery, turnip or kohlrabi strips to use as "pushers" rather than the usual white roll.

The curry sauce should be barely cooked with the vegetables still crunchy to the teeth, as in Chinese foods.

CURRY SAUCE

¼ cup butter
½ cup chopped onions
¼ cup chopped celery
¼ cup chopped bell pepper (include the seeds and inner membrane)

Optional:

1″, or smaller, piece grated ginger root
1 large diced apple (unpeeled)
Fresh coconut, grated (reserve its milk, if available)
1 small clove garlic, crushed

Melt the butter over a low heat (*don't let it brown*), and add above ingredients. As soon as the vegetables have become golden and softened a bit, add a mixture of:

2 rounded teaspoons arrowroot
1 teaspoon curry powder
Seasoning salt, to taste
½ cup vegetable broth *or* soup stock
2 additional cups broth or stock

This should be mixed well and added to vegetables with 2 additional cups of stock and the coconut milk. Heat and stir until the arrowroot has cleared and thickened your gravy. It is now ready to serve over brown rice.

Arrange your serving table with a choice of:

Cooked brown rice	Sliced fresh papaya
Salad greens	Grated fresh coconut
Sesame seeds	Diced fresh pineapple
Sunflower seeds	Chutney
Diced tomatoes	Diced raw mushrooms
Diced green onions	Grated ginger sparingly
Chopped almonds	Diced green pepper

Even the most finicky eater should be able to find a satisfying combination among these foods, which appeal to vegetarians and carnivores, raw food and cooked food aficionados alike.

MUSHROOM SPAGHETTI SAUCE

1 onion, chopped
1 good-sized garlic clove, pressed
1 cup sliced, fresh mushrooms
1 green pepper
1 teaspoon kelp
1 teaspoon oregano
½ teaspoon basil
¼ teaspoon cayenne
Sea salt, to taste
1 to 2 tablespoons olive oil
1 #2½ can tomato puree
1 6-oz. can tomato paste
1 bay leaf
½ cup chopped pecans
Artichoke or buckwheat flour spaghetti noodles
(if you are unable to find spaghetti squash)

Warm the onion, garlic, mushrooms, green pepper, and the seasonings (except bay leaf) in the oil. Add the tomato products and the bay leaf; bring this to a boil and then simmer for 5 minutes. Add pecans just before serving. Serve over your cooked noodles.

Legumes

Legumes—dried navy, red, kidney, pinto, great northern, garbanzo, black, soy, and lima beans and split peas and lentils—very frequently make up a large portion of the vegetarian main dish. They seem to be good sources of abscisic acid, are easy to prepare, are easily digested if prepared as suggested, and are therefore appropriate *for all diets*

Soaking: Boil the dried legumes for 10 minutes and allow them to sit, soaking off the heat in a covered pan for 1 hour. This will tenderize them, making their digestion less difficult.

Cooking: Cooking takes place after the 1 hour soaking period is completed. Continue cooking the legumes until tender.

Pureeing: To make a soup base legumes may be pureed in the blender after they are cooked. Create a thick or thin base by adding the desired amount of liquid.

BASIC BEAN PREPARATION

> **1 cup beans (pinto, kidney, garbanzos, most beans)**
> **Boiling water**
> **1 or 2 bay leaves**

Wash the beans, removing any broken bits or foreign matter. Cover them with boiling water, add the bay leaves, and cook ½ hour. Remove from heat and let the mixture sit 1 to 2 hours, covered. Return to low heat and cook 1½ to 3 hours, or until tender. Test the beans with a fork. Save the cooking water, as it contains valuable nutrients and should be used.

CROCK POT BEANS MEXICAN STYLE

> **1 lb. or about 2½ cups beans (pink, red, pinto, or kidney)**
> **Boiling water, enough to cover**

Stir the beans into the boiling water and boil for 10 minutes. Remove from the heat and allow to soak for 1 to 2 hours, then drain and proceed with the recipe. Transfer the presoaked beans to your crock pot, adding:

> 4 cups water
> 1 teaspoon herb seasoned salt
> 1 to 2 teaspoons chili powder
> 2 cloves garlic, sliced
> 1 large onion, chopped
> ½ teaspoon oregano

Cover crock pot and turn to high, near boiling, for 2 hours. Lower the heat for 6 to 8 hours.

Suggestion: 1 lb. fresh tomatoes cut into eighths may be added during the last hour of cooking.

MEXICAN REFRIED BEANS

> 1 cup cooked pinto beans
> ¼ cup chopped onion (optional)
> Butter

Melt the butter in a skillet, adding the onion. Place the pinto beans on top, mashing and stirring as they heat through. Serve with corn tostadas.

LENTILS AND ONIONS

> 1 medium onion, chopped
> 2 cups sliced mushrooms
> ¼ cup butter
> 2 cups cooked lentils
> 1 teaspoon herb seasoned salt
> 1 teaspoon kelp, to taste, or papaya seed pepper, to taste

Lightly sauté the onions and mushrooms in the butter. Add the remaining ingredients and serve.

LENTIL PATTIES

2 cups cooked lentils
⅓ cup chopped celery
⅓ cup chopped onions
⅓ cup grated carrot
½ cup ground sunflower or pumpkin seeds
½ cup ground cashews
1 teaspoon herb seasoned salt
1 teaspoon thyme
½ cup bread crumbs (homemade or whole grain)

Mix all ingredients thoroughly, adding the bread crumbs as needed, to form patties. Place the patties onto an oiled cookie sheet and heat in a moderate oven only long enough to firm and warm. Serve.

BRAZIL NUT ROAST

2 cups cooked lentils
1 cup cooked brown rice
1 cup cooked garbanzos blended with ½ cup vegetable broth
¾ cup chopped Brazil nuts
2 teaspoons Selenium yeast
1 teaspoon herb seasoned salt (sea salt base)
  or ½ teaspoon dried herbs mixed with
  ½ teaspoon sea salt

Mix lentils and rice with blended garbanzos. Stir in the chopped nuts, yeast, herbed salt, or herbs and salt mixture. Place in buttered baking dish and bake for 1 hour at 325° F.

CASHEW ROAST

1 cup cashews
1 small clove garlic
1 cup garbanzo cooking water

1½ cups cooked garbanzos
2 cups cooked brown rice
1 cup grated carrot
1 teaspoon herb seasoned salt
½ teaspoon kelp
1 cup onions sautéed in a small amount of butter

Blend the cashews, garlic, and garbanzo cooking water in the blender. Add garbanzos and blend again. Mix with the brown rice, grated carrots, herb seasoned salt, kelp, and sautéed onions. Place in a buttered baking dish and bake 1 hour at 325° F.

KIDNEY BEAN BURGERS

2 tablespoons butter
¼ cup scissor-snipped chives or onion tops
¼ cup scissor-snipped parsley
2½ cups cooked kidney beans

Melt the butter in a skillet. Add the chives, parsley, and cooked beans. Mash and stir the beans with chives and parsley, cooking over a very low heat until thick enough to shape into burgers. Serve with lemon if desired.

GRANDMOTHER'S BEAN SOUP

1 lb. or 2⅓ cups navy beans, white beans, *or* split peas
2 quarts boiling water

Stir the beans into the boiling water and cook 10 minutes. Remove from the heat and soak 1 to 2 hours. Transfer to a crock pot and add:

1 teaspoon sea salt
10 papaya seeds
1 cup chopped outer stalks of celery with the root
2 onions, sliced
2 bay leaves
4 large carrots, sliced

Place the lid on the crock pot and reheat on high, then turn to low for 8 to 10 hours.

Fermented and Cultured Foods

FIZZY APPLE

1 gallon raw apple juice
1/16 teaspoon baker's yeast

Pour off ½ cup of juice from the gallon jug. Discard ¼ cup and mix ¼ cup with the baker's yeast. Return this mixture to the gallon jug of apple juice and replace the pressure seal lid, or just barely catch the screw lid. When the lid has blown off several times (it won't overflow, the lid just pops off), and little bubbles, like champagne bubbles, are traveling up the sides of the bottle, it is ready to refrigerate.

The first stage tastes like apple soda pop, the next stage like champagne, the next like beer, and finally, apple cider vinegar. Try to make just enough to use during the first two stages. Sometimes, raw apple juice will get fizzy in the refrigerator all by itself if left long enough. This keeps at least a week in the refrigerator. Always save a starter for your next batch!

BEET RELISH

3 large beets
1/3 cup honey

Juice 1 beet (or more if necessary). The juice must cover the grated vegetable. Grate the other 2 beets. Add the honey to the beet juice and cover the grated beets with this mixture. It is most important that the juice cover the beets thoroughly. Place the beets-and-juice mixture in a glass bowl, covering it with cheesecloth and allowing to ferment 36 to 48 hours at room temperature. Chill and serve. Makes 2 to 3 cups.

Suggestions: Add ⅓ cup apple cider vinegar or lemon juice to taste, and serve as pickled beets; *or* dilute the relish with water and add tomatoes, green onions, etc., serving as a borscht; *or* serve diluted as a raw beet soup; *or* use ½ tablespoon vegetable gelatin to ⅛ cup water. Add this mixture, whirling it in the blender, to ¾ cup of the juice, and let thicken to egg-white consistency. Add the grated beets and refrigerate until firm.

RAW SAUERKRAUT

2 heads red or green cabbage (naturally grown if possible)

Utensils:

1 crock or glass bowl
Glass lid *or* ceramic plate without painted design
    (painted design will dissolve into fermented cabbage, and
    it is toxic)

Peel off the outside leaves of the cabbage and save. Shred the heads as finely as possible to provide the necessary juice for fermentation. Place the shredded cabbage and all its juice in your crock or glass bowl. Lay the whole leaves over the top. Place your plate or lid on top of the leaves (lid *must* be smaller than crock so as to move downwards as the fermentation takes place). Fill a ½-gallon jar with water, using this as a weight to set on top of the plate. The cabbage will ferment in 5 to 7 days and lasts indefinitely. Note: Raw sauerkraut ferments at room temperature

CASHEW COTTAGE CHEESE

Cashews
Water

Soak cashews overnight in enough water to cover. Blend the next morning, and leave at room temperature for 1 day. It will resemble cottage cheese.

CONDIMENTS AND SAUCES

HERB SEASONED SALT

⅛ cup sea salt
⅛ cup kelp
1 tablespoon dried parsley
⅛ teaspoon dill powder
¼ teaspoon onion powder
¼ teaspoon garlic powder
½ teaspoon paprika
⅛ teaspoon basil and/or oregano
Toasted sesame seed, ground to taste

Mix ingredients together and use in place of salt. Experiment to find the flavors you enjoy.

PAPAYA SEED PEPPER

Seeds from a fresh papaya

Rinse the pulp off the seeds, and lay the clean seeds on a paper towel to dry, perhaps in your oven. They should be thoroughly dry in several days. Store them in a glass jar in the refrigerator until you are ready to use them. Grind them in an electric seed mill or pepper mill. Use in place of black pepper.

Suggestions: Ground papaya seeds are a delicious addition to fresh salad dressing. In moderation, papaya seeds are a digestive aid. In excess they are difficult to handle.

SESAME YEAST SPREAD

2 ozs. sesame seeds, finely ground
1 tablespoon Dr. Jensen's Vegetable Powder
⅓ cup water
1 tablespoon nutritional yeast

Blend all the ingredients and serve on zucchini, cucumber, or carrot rounds. Resembles the taste of tuna fish.

HUMUS—GARBANZO PUREE

> 2 cups cooked garbanzos
> 1 large garlic clove, minced
> 2 tablespoons tahini (sesame butter)
> Juice of ½ lemon
> 1 teaspoon ascorbic acid crystals
> ½ teaspoon olive oil
> Sesame salt to taste

Puree all ingredients in the blender until creamy. Serve as a spread on carrots, celery, or other raw vegetables.

HOMEMADE RAW CATSUP

> 1 lb. tomatoes
> ¼ cup olive oil
> ½ onion, chopped
> 1 green onion, chopped
> 1 tablespoon honey
> 1 tablespoon lemon juice
> ½ teaspoon kelp or sea salt, to taste
> ¼ teaspoon oregano, basil, other desired herbs
> 1 very small garlic clove

Blend. Water can be drained from the blended mixture to get a thicker consistency. Keep in the refrigerator.

RAW MEXICAN "SALSA"

> 4 tomatoes
> 1 onion, chopped coarsely
> Chili peppers, chopped (to taste;
>   often *just* ½ small pepper is enough)

1 teaspoon herb seasoned salt
1 red bell pepper, chopped
1 small clove garlic

Blend all ingredients and store in the refrigerator. This mixes well with Eggless Mayonnaise. It also goes well with vegetable salads and fish recipes (for Non-Strict Diets).

COMFREY CASHEW SAUCE

½ cup cashews
½ cup water
2 chopped comfrey leaves (large, mature leaves)
1 small garlic clove
1 teaspoon kelp
Herbed seasoning, if desired

Blend to desired consistency and serve over vegetables, salads, or serve warm as a gravy.

RAW MUSHROOM SAUCE

2 tablespoons butter
1 large green onion, finely chopped
1 cup sliced fresh mushrooms
¼ teaspoon oregano
1 tablespoon tahini (sesame butter)
1 cup Almond Milk, page 164
1 small clove garlic, pressed
¼ teaspoon herb seasoned salt
Dr. Jensen's Broth Seasoning, to taste

Warm the butter (*do not brown*) and lightly warm the onion and mushrooms with the oregano. (The mushrooms may be blended if desired.) Remove from the heat, cover, and let sit. Blend together the tahini, Almond Milk, garlic, and remaining seasonings. Add more tahini to thicken if desired. Warm this sauce with the buttered onion and mushrooms.

TARTAR SAUCE

1 cup Eggless Mayonnaise, page 199
4 tablespoons lemon juice
¼ teaspoon ground dill seeds
½ cup diced cucumber
1 green onion, very finely chopped (green end also)
⅛ cup minced parsley

Mix all ingredients. Let chill together briefly and serve.

HOMEMADE TOMATO SAUCE

6 large tomatoes
2 cups water
1 medium onion, chopped
1 teaspoon honey, raw
1 teaspoon sea salt (optional)
1 teaspoon kelp
1 large garlic clove, pressed
1 teaspoon each: sweet basil, oregano, parsley

Cook the tomatoes alone over medium heat for 5 minutes. Add all remaining ingredients and cook for 10 more minutes. Remove from heat. Strain off most of the liquid and puree in the blender until smooth.

SESAME SALT

This delicious seasoning can halve your salt intake.

Herb seasoned salt
(containing no preservatives, chemicals or additives;
read labels *carefully*)
Toasted sesame seeds

Grind up equal amounts of ingredients and mix. (Small nut mills are perfect for this.) To retain freshness, grind only 1 week's worth at a time.

RAW BEET SAUCE

2 medium beets, shredded
2 medium small carrots, shredded
2 oz. water
1 oz. oil
1 tablespoon honey
Juice of ½ to 1 lemon *or* lime

Place the beets, carrots, and water in a blender and blend. While blending, slowly add the oil in a thin stream. Remove from the blender, and pour into a bowl. Add the honey and citrus juice to taste. Serve over shredded beets and carrots or zucchini.

HOLLANDAISE SAUCE

¼ cup Eggless Mayonnaise, page 199
¹⁄₁₆ teaspoon dry mustard
½ teaspoon raw honey
A dash of garlic
A dash of sea salt

Blend all ingredients and serve with vegetables.

RAW APPLE, CURRANT AND PAPAYA CHUTNEY

1 apple, diced into small cubes
1 green pepper, sliced thinly
1 clove garlic
Water
1 small papaya, diced
1 tablespoon lemon juice
¼ teaspoon sea salt
¼ teaspoon ginger
¾ teaspoon paprika
⅓ cup currants
2 tablespoons raw honey
½ teaspoon cinnamon

Place the apple, green pepper, garlic and enough water to cover in the blender. Blend until the vegetables are chopped fine. Drain off the water and place in a bowl. Blend the papaya alone. Add all ingredients, combine, and chill before serving.

SPICY APPLE BUTTER

  1 recipe of Homemade Applesauce, page 231
  1½ teaspoons ground cinnamon*
  ¾ teaspoon ground cloves*
  ¼ teaspoon allspice

Mix all the ingredients, pouring off any juice that separates.

SNACKS AND DESSERTS

The best snacks are raw vegetables and fruits (naturally grown and fully ripe), nuts, and seeds. Always save the pulp and seeds from such fruits as apples and watermelon, because they can be blended and strained to make an excellent natural protein drink. Eat the seeds of grapes.

Always eat the skins and seeds of your fruit. Peel the skin of an orange with a potato peeler, so that you can eat more of the white pulp just beneath it. The pulp is full of bioflavinoids, which enhance the metabolism of vitamin C.

Shell your own nuts to be sure they are fresh. Cashews are an excellent source of abscisins, so eat them freely. Also eat lots of almonds, Brazil nuts, hazelnuts, macadamia nuts, pecans, pistachios, and walnuts. To put some fun into your snacking, find a good nutcracker and use it often. A good nutcracker can make eating nuts less tedious.

---

*The cinnamon and cloves can be freshly ground in a seed mill from a cinnamon stick and whole cloves.

Use your food processor to make nut butters to spread on bread and toast or eat with snacks.

There are a few desserts in this section, meant for special occasions, whose ingredients include natural sugars. But in general *avoid all sugar* in your diet, even in snacks and desserts. The *P. Cryptocides* microbe seems to thrive on it!

ARROWROOT PUDDING

Arrowroot puddings are simply made and an excellent source of calcium. *Two tablespoons of arrowroot will thicken 1 cup of liquid.* Create your own favorite flavor and enjoy whenever the need for a comforting and familiar snack-food is desired.

BASIC PUDDING

> **5 tablespoons arrowroot**
> **½ cup water**
> **1½ cups boiling water**
> **½ teaspoon honey**
> **Juice of ½ lemon**
> **1 teaspoon grated lemon rind**

Stir the arrowroot into the ½ cup of water. Add this mixture to the 1½ cups water that have been brought to a boil, stirring over the heat and allowing it to clear and thicken. Remove from heat and add the remaining ingredients.

BASIC PUDDING
WITH CHERRY CONCENTRATE

Follow directions for Basic Pudding. After removing the pudding from heat add:

> **1½ tablespoons cherry concentrate**

Serve with a nut cream if desired.

APPLE ARROWROOT PUDDING

5 tablespoons arrowroot
½ cup water
1½ cups apple juice
½ teaspoon honey
1 teaspoon grated lemon rind
1 large apple, finely diced
Cinnamon

Stir the arrowroot into the ½ cup water. Bring apple juice to a boil. Add arrowroot mixture to the apple juice, stirring over the heat and allowing it to clear and thicken. Remove from the heat and add remaining ingredients.

CAROB PUDDING

5 tablespoons arrowroot
3 tablespoons carob powder
½ cup water
1½ cups boiling water
½ teaspoon honey
1 tablespoon grated orange or dried tangerine rind

Stir the arrowroot and carob powder into the ½ cup of water. Add this mixture to the 1½ cups water that have been brought to a boil, stirring over the heat and allowing it to clear and thicken. Remove from the heat and add remaining ingredients. Serve with a nut cream if desired.

FROZEN CAROB BANANAS

Bananas
⅓ cup carob powder
⅓ cup soy-milk powder
⅓ cup raw cream
1 tablespoon honey

1 tablespoon vanilla
Nuts (optional)

Slice bananas 1" thick or peel and leave whole. Place on wooden skewers or toothpicks, arrange on a cookie sheet, and freeze. Mix other ingredients together and when the bananas are firmly frozen, spoon the sauce over them. (You may need more cream if the mixture is too thick). Sprinkle on chopped nuts if you wish. Return, well wrapped, to the freezer until needed.

Suggestion: For parties you may find it quicker to place the carob topping in an icing gun and put a rosette on each slice.

BUTTERSCOTCH PUDDING

¼ cup chopped figs
¼ cup pitted and chopped dates
⅛ teaspoon Malt Sweetner
1 teaspoon grated lemon rind
5 tablespoons arrowroot
½ cup water
1½ cups boiling water

Blend the figs and dates with enough water to make a thick spread; set aside. Add the arrowroot to the ½ cup of water, stirring until smooth. Add this arrowroot mixture to 1½ cups of boiling water, stirring it over the heat and allowing it to clear and thicken; then add the fig-date mixture. Remove from the heat and add the remaining ingredients, serving with a nut cream if desired.

Suggestion: If you wish to keep the fig-date mixture raw, you may add it *after* the pudding has cooled.

PINEAPPLE ARROWROOT PUDDING

5 tablespoons arrowroot
½ cup water
1½ cups pineapple juice
Fresh pineapple chunks (optional)

Stir the arrowroot into the ½ cup water. Bring the pineapple juice to a boil, then add the arrowroot mixture to it. Stir over the heat, allowing liquid to clear and thicken. Remove from the heat and add remaining ingredients.

BANANAS AND AVOCADO

6 bananas
½ cup fresh orange juice
Whipped cream
½ cup ground pumpkin seeds *or* walnuts
Lettuce *or* other greens
1 avocado

Dip the bananas in orange juice. Cover with whipped cream, and sprinkle with ground seeds or nuts. Serve on greens with sliced avocado.

NATURAL FRUIT GELATIN

Place 1 tablespoon of gelatin or 3 tablespoons agar-agar and ½ cup of your favorite fruit juice in a saucepan and bring to a boil. Pour into 1 pint of fresh juice in mixing bowl. Put in the refrigerator until solidified or, when cool and partially set, shredded vegetables or chopped fruits may be added.

APPLESAUCE PIE

Seed Nut Crust, page 233
Homemade Applesauce, page 231
Whipped cream (optional)
Nuts (optional)

Make the Seed Nut Crust, patting it into a glass pie dish. Prepare your Homemade Applesauce, spooning it into your crust. Top with whipped cream and chopped nuts, if desired.

HOMEMADE APPLESAUCE

Pineapple juice, approx. ⅓ cup
(frozen or fresh)
1 teaspoon vitamin C powder
(to retard browning of apples)
4 or more apples, quartered
Dash of cinnamon (optional)
Dash of nutmeg (optional)

Place the juice and the vitamin C powder in your blender. Add several apple quarters at a time, turning blender on and off until a puree is developed. Cinnamon and nutmeg may then be added. Use immediately.

Suggestions: The applesauce may be frozen if it will not be used immediately. Do not peel the apples unless they are unnaturally grown.

APPLE PIE

Seed Nut Crust (omitting butter), page 233
Apples, sliced and dipped in pineapple juice
½ teaspoon vegetable gelatin
¼ cup apple juice
¾ cup apple juice
Cinnamon, to taste

Shape ½ of the crust recipe into a pie dish. Cover with sliced apples that have been dipped into pineapple juice (this prevents discoloring). Freeze. Place ½ teaspoon gelatin in ¼ cup apple juice and melt gently over hot water. Blend together remaining ¾ cups apple juice and cinnamon, and then add the gelatin mixture into the blender whirlpool. Pour the blended ingredients over the frozen apple pie. This gives the frozen apples a "cooked" texture upon thawing and will congeal the apple juice as well as thicken the crust. It should look like a baked apple pie. Top with remaining ½ pie crust.

PRUNE WHIP

2 cups dry prunes that have been soaked overnight
Prune soak water (enough to cover the prunes)
¼ cup cashew butter, or to desired consistency
1 teaspoon honey
½ teaspoon pure vanilla

Remove the pits from the soaked prunes, then crack open the pit
shells, and remove the kernels. They will be used with the recipe,
as all fruit kernels are high in abscisins. Blend the prunes with
a little soak water. Add the cashew butter, remaining soak water,
honey, and vanilla. Blend until smooth, adding more water or
cashew butter to adjust to the consistency you desire. Serve with
the kernels ground on top.

RAW FUDGE

½ cup butter *or* ½ cup almond butter
1 tablespoon vanilla
½ cup Almond Milk, page 164
1 cup carob powder
1 cup arrowroot powder
1 cup grated fresh coconut
1 cup coarsely ground walnuts

Cream the butter with the vanilla, adding the Almond Milk
slowly.

Mix the carob powder with the arrowroot powder. Combine
this mixture with the creamed butter, adding more Almond Milk
if necessary.

Lastly, add the coconut and walnuts. Press the entire mixture
into a buttered square dish and chill (or roll into balls and chill).

Serve cut into squares.

Butter, almonds, carob, and walnuts are all abscisic acid
sources. The arrowroot and carob are both rich sources of calcium
and trace minerals. Coconut adds valuable fibers. This gives you
"raw fudge" with no added sweeteners.

APRICOT BALLS

1 cup apricots (unsulfured and sundried) and the kernels
from their pits (de-cyanided)
½ cup almonds
½ lb. coconut, fresh
1 teaspoon lemon juice
1 heaping teaspoon ascorbic acid

Chop together in your blender or food chopper the apricots,
almonds, de-cyanided apricot kernels, and coconut. Add the
lemon juice and ascorbic acid, shape into balls, and if desired,
roll in ground almonds or leftover ground coconut.

SEED NUT CRUST
(For Non-Strict Diet)

⅔ cup ground cashews
⅓ cup ground sesame seeds
⅓ cup soft butter
½ teaspoon cinnamon
½ teaspoon nutmeg

Mix ingredients until crumbly. Pat into pie pan or tart cups, as
needed.

GLOSSARY

ABSCISIC ACID.   An analog of vitamin A, the plant hormone known as dormin responsible for hibernation of seeds and nuts. Retards growth of cells and destroys CG (choriogonadotropin).

ACID-FAST.   Capable of retaining certain red dyes, such as carbol fushin, after decolorization (washing) with acid alcohol on a glass microscope slide.

ADENOCARCINOMA.   Glandular carcinoma.

ADRENALECTOMY.   Surgical removal of part or all of an adrenal gland (near each kidney).

ADJUVANT.   A drug added to an antigen to hasten or increase the action of a principal ingredient.

AGGLUTINATE.   To unite or cause to adhere.

ANALOG.   Counterfeit of a real vitamin that is made to "fool" the cancer cell in its requirement for the essential vitamin; the cancer incorporates the counterfeit into the cell and is killed.

ANTIBODY.   A protein substance in the body which incites immunity by reacting with an antigen.

ANTIGEN.   A biological substance, such as a vaccine or foreign protein, that produces an immunological response by producing antibodies.

ATTENUATE.   To make less virulent; to weaken.

AUTOGENOUS VACCINE.   A suspension of *Progenitor Cryptocides* that has been killed and suspended in a dilute solution of phenol (as a preservative) or other bacteriostat. An autogenous vaccine is made from each patient's own culture. It is administered in standard amounts in ascending doses in order to increase immunity.

AXILLA.   The armpit.

BACILLUS.   Rod-shaped bacterium.

BACTERIA.   Any of numerous microscopic, spherical, rod-shaped, or spiral organisms. May be nonpathogenic or pathogenic.

BCG VACCINE.   *Bacillus Calmette-Guérin*, attenuated vaccine of bovine tubercule bacillus used to vaccinate against tuberculosis.

CG (CHORIOGONADOTROPIN).   A mammalian hormone produced in the trophoblast of the placenta. *Progenitor Cryptocides* is present in spermatozoa, bone marrow, placenta, and cancer cells where it produces CG. This hormone protects the fetus and the cancer cell from destruction by the immune defenses of the body.

CHEMOTHERAPY.   Treatment of cancer with certain chemicals that interfere with cell division and affect not only the cancer cells but all young and dividing cells of the body, such as blood cells. Chemotherapy alone may destroy immunity if given too long and too intensely. It is not usually curative except in rare instances.

COCCOIDAL. Resembling a micrococcus, a type of bacteria which is spherical or oval in form.

COLLAGEN DISEASE. A disease in which all the connective tissues of the body are involved and in which such tissues may have a common origin in cell malformation, such as arthritis, hardening of the arteries, rheumatic fever, etc.

COMPLEMENT. A substance in blood serum and plasma that in combination with antibodies destroys bacteria, foreign cells, and other antigens.

CULTURE. A purposeful growth of microorganisms for scientific study.

CYTO-. Pertaining to the cell.

CYTOPLASM. Protoplasm.

DARK-FIELD MICROSCOPE. A microscope in which light is reflected from the specimen on the slide up through the eyepiece, causing the specimen, such as microbes or blood cells on the glass slide, to have a bright appearance against a dark background. Living, unstained specimens are used and may be projected upon a television screen, demonstrating their motility. Used for examining living blood and microbes.

ECHOGRAM. An ultrasound technique using echoes or reverberations to detect the presence of tumors and lesions.

ELECTRON MICROSCOPE. A microscope capable of magnifying several hundred thousand times; however, the area it can observe is very small. It is primarily a research instrument.

ENDOMETRIUM. The mucous membrane lining the inner surface of the uterus.

ENZYME. A protein or other substance secreted by certain body cells that induces chemical changes in other substances, itself apparently remaining unchanged in the process.

EPITHELIAL. Pertaining to or composed of the layer of cells forming the epidermis, or surface layer of the skin; also applies to the outer layer of the lining of organs.

FILTRATE. A liquid that has been passed through a filter.

FUNGOID BACILLUS. A bacillus having the appearance of a fungus, a vegetable cellular organism that subsists on organic matter.

GAMMA GLOBULIN. A suspension of the immune bodies from plasma. It is nonspecific but protects against many infections, such as measles and hepatitis. It has been shown to give passive immunity to cancer patients.

GLOBULIN. A simple protein soluble only in neutral salt solutions, concerned with the transport of antibodies to combat infection.

GRANULOMA. A granular tumor or growth, usually of lymphoid and epithelial cells.

HODGKIN'S DISEASE. A chronic infectious disease that produces enlargement of lymphoid tissue, spleen, liver, and sometimes kidneys. It is one form of lymphoma.

HYPOPHYSECTOMY. Excision of the pituitary gland.

IMMUNITY. The condition of resistance to a specific protein, such as viruses, bacteria, and toxins. Immunity protects the individual from the diseased state against which he or she has been immunized, such as tetanus, polio, and measles.

IMMUNOSUPPRESSION. A state of lowered immunity induced by poor nutrition, disease, chemicals, radiation, chemotherapy, trauma, and debility that causes susceptibility to infection.

INTERSTITIAL. Placed or lying between; occupying space between the central parts of an organ.

LAPAROTOMY. The surgical opening of the abdomen; an abdominal operation.

LEUKOSIS. The presence of an abnormal number of leukocytes in the blood.

LEUKOCYTE. A white blood corpuscle.

LIGHT MICROSCOPE. A microscope in which light passes directly through the specimen, which is usually not alive but fixed or stained; the specimen is projected in color against a light background. Used for examining cultures, blood, tissues, and smears.

LYMPHOCYTE. A white blood cell produced in lymphoid tissue.

LYMPHOMA. A lymphoid tissue tumor.

MEDIASTINUM. The folds of the pleura and intervening space between the right and left lung.

MESODERMAL. Pertaining to the middle layer of cells in the germinal membrane of an embryo.

METASTASIS, METASTASIZE. Movement of cells or bacterium from one part of the body to another, or the change in location of a disease from one organ to part of another; to invade by *metastasis*. (Plural: *metastases*.)

MICROORGANISM. A microscopic plant or animal.

MICROBE. A pathogenic bacterium.

MICRON. A millionth of a meter.

MORPHOLOGY. The form and structure of an organism considered as a whole.

MYCELIA. The vegetative part of the fungus, being composed of one or more filiamentous elements.

MYCO-. Funguslike.

MYCOBACTERIUM. Any of several rod-shaped aerobic bacteria of the genus *Mycobacterium*, certain species of which are pathogenic for human beings and animals.

NEOPLASIA. The formation and growth of new tissue; tumor growth.

NITRAZINE PAPER. A test paper treated with a chemical to indicate whether the urine or any fluid is acid or alkaline. It has a comparison scale or indicator attached. Over pH 7 is alkaline and under pH 7 is acid.

-OMA. A suffix denoting a tumor.

OMENTUM. An apronlike fold in the abdomen enclosing the bowels.

ONCOLOGY, ONCOLOGIST. The branch of medical science dealing with tumors; a medical doctor specializing in cancer.

OOPHORECTOMY. Excision of an ovary.

ORCHIECTOMY. Excision of a testicle.

PARASITIZATION. To live on a host, as a parasite.

PEPTONES. Any of a class of diffusible, soluble substances into which proteins are converted by partial hydrolysis.

PERIAORTIC. Around or alongside the aorta.

PERICARDIUM. The sac enclosing the heart and the roots of the great blood vessels.

PERITONEUM. The serous membrane reflected over the viscera and lining the abdominal cavity.

PETRI DISH. A shallow, circular, glass or plastic dish with a loose-fitting cover, used for culturing bacteria and other microorganisms.

PHAGOCYTOSIS. Ingestion and digestion of bacteria and particles by a white blood cell called a *phagocyte*.

PLEOMORPHIC. Having many forms.

PPD (PURIFIED PROTEIN DERIVATIVE). An extract of the tubercle bacillus used to skin test a person to determine the presence or absence of antibodies to tuberculosis. A positive test, consisting of redness and swelling, indicates immunity and also previous infection.

RADIATION. Treatment of cancer by destroying the cells with ionizing radiation. This process destroys not only the cancer but healthy cells as well; it causes long term deterioration of tissues, such as atrophy, loss of vascularity, poor healing, and skin changes.

RAYNAUD'S SYNDROME (or Raynaud's Disease). A severe vascular disorder causing disturbances in the circulation of the extremities.

SCAN. A radioisotopic survey of the body or a portion of the body, used as a diagnostic tool for the detection of disease.

SCLERODERMA. The prefix *sclero-* means *hard*. *Scleroderma* is a disease of the skin and internal organs causing rigidity, thickening, and malfunction.

SKIN TESTS. These consist of intradermal tests for tuberculosis and focal infection, as an indication of immune state. Performed on both forearms.

SPLENECTOMY. Excision of the spleen.

SYSTEMIC. Invading the whole body rather than one of its parts.

TROPHOBLAST. The outer layer of placenta cells which communicates with the uterus and regulates nutrition of the fetus.

VIRUS. Any of a group of ultramicroscopic, infectious agents that reproduce only in living cells.

ZYGOTE. A cell produced by the union of two gametes, in humans an ovum and sperm.

EPILOGUE

As this book goes to press it is gratifying to note that our findings have been further supported by new research reported in such prestigious journals as *Scientific American* ("A Vector for Introducing New Genes into Plants," June, 1983, p. 51) and *Lancet* ("Vitamin A and Retinoids," April 16, 1983, p. 860). *The New England Journal of Medicine* has also recently published a report on the role vitamin A and the retinoids might have in treating bone cancer.

Furthermore, the popular press has begun to report on the relationship between genetic engineering, biological intervention and the cure of cancer (e.g., *The New York Times Magazine*, October 24, 1982, and *Reader's Digest*, March, 1983), and recently it seems as if every week there is a new announcement about "optimistic" results of certain tests having to do with a "virus-like" microorganism.

Perhaps even most exciting of all has been the appearance of an article in *The New England Journal of Medicine* (June 16, 1983, p. 1476), describing tests on a 43-year-old male homosexual with Kaposi's sarcoma. During carbolfushin staining of the spindle cells of the tumor, the researcher reports, "Surprisingly, abundant acid-fast microorganisms were demonstrated..." This is highly encouraging because over the years we have cultured lesions of a number of cases of Kaposi's sarcoma, and invariably we have found the acid-fast P.C. microbe. This work also was recently confirmed by Dr. Alan Cantwell of Kaiser Permanante Hospital in the July 1983 issue of *Cutis*.

The onset of a mycobacterial disease almost always leads to a loss of immunity. We believe that the effective treatment of AIDS can be instituted by the same immunotherapy program that we customarily use in the treatment of cancer. The P.C. microbe's transmissivity in human sperm; the immunity breakdown; the fact that homosexual men with AIDS usually develop cancer; the fact that homosexual women seldom contract AIDS; the fact, as reported by the National Cancer Institute, that it seems to be the passive partner in the homosexual transmission of sperm who contracts AIDS—all this hints at the need for further research into the activity and causative relationship of the hidden killer, *Progenitor Cryptocides*. We definitely feel that investigation into the immunotherapy of Kaposi's Syndrome is in order.

While it continues to grieve me that millions of dollars are still being spent on testing cures in rats and mice while I have been curing *human beings* for fifteen years, most of the thinking scientific community will now admit that immunotherapy, based on the molecular structure of the cell, is the hope of the future. The standard treatments with radiation and chemotherapy are a shotgun approach based on destruction of cells instead of regulation and control of the neoplastic process.

At a recent conference on molecular immunology at Stanford University, two cases of recovery from acute leukemia with the use of hybridoma were reported. This is a process in which a patient's own tissues were used to immunize a mouse and then the mouse's immunized spleen cells were hybridized with cancer cells, and then the immune hybrids cultured and finally administered to the patient as a vaccine. This is almost exactly what we are doing in San Diego, except that if a universal antigen such as our P. Cryptocides or one of its derivatives were used, then the antibodies would not need to be specific to a certain type of tumor, but could be used in the universal treatment of all cancers. Such studies, in which we are participating, are now in progress, using certain immunity-producing human cell components and thereby eliminating the need to use mouse cells for hybridization.

Also, the current research into "oncogenes" and the DNA and RNA molecules having to do with the genetic mutations of cells that seem to cause cancerous growth, appears to be related to the production of CG in the cell and the growth of the P.C. microbe. Since all tumor cells contain CG, which acts as a shield against immune bodies, then the neutralization of CG could be helpful. I have proved that abscisic acid is a part of the vitamin A group and has a profound influence on the growth of cells. In the test tube it inhibits the production of CG. It also appears that two enzymes in the human liver, called xanthine oxidase and tyrosinase, convert vitamin A to the abscisins, hence are extremely important in the neutralization of CG and the ultimate remission of cancer.

I am confident that all my findings will be universally corroborated and that my treatment methods, or close variations thereof, will eventually become the prevalent treatment of cancer. My results have been so consistently remarkable over the course of three decades that serious researchers and clinical experimenters cannot venture in any other direction. Prestigious institutions around the nation—Princeton, Duke, University of California, et al.—are already reexamining the papers I published in the '40s and '50s, and my experiments are being replicated.

A cure is *now* at hand. In a generation or sooner, cancer will be as rare a disease as smallpox or polio. But effecting that cure is at the same time simple and complex. It is as simple as avoiding the superinfection produced by the bacterial form of the P.C. microbe—in our food chain and in the precipitating carcinogenic factors of many types in our environment.

It is as complex as convincing the politicians involved (not necessarily those who seek public office) that immunization at birth is the first step.

We can survive on this planet only by understanding what is happening within the sixty billion cells that make up an adult human being. When I recently watched a presentation of our future in outer space I was profoundly struck by the fact that our fragility as the human species in the totality of the universe was ignored. What is the adaptability of our protoplasm? What are our biological needs and how can they be met in space over the eons of time? The infinitude of the molecular spaces within our own bodies matches that of the outermost complexities of the universe.

But what are we to do *now?* I propose that all infants be immunized at birth. BCG is reasonably effective, but the real agent, the *P. Cryptocides*, should be used. We should also eliminate cancer from our food chain by vaccinating cattle and chickens, and feeding our food animals with uncontaminated materials. We should immunize our pets to stop cross-infection. We should control the chemicalization of our fruit trees, plants and vegetables by promoting the use of natural deterrents. We should promote, *not criticize,* diets that are vegetarian or composed mostly of natural foods and raw vegetables. We should assume greater control of toxic materials used by industry and control the petrochemicals in our enviroment.

Virginia Livingston-Wheeler, M.D.
La Jolla, California
July 22, 1983

APPENDIX

TEN CASES I WISH AN INDEPENDENT MEDICAL PANEL WOULD INVESTIGATE

All these cases except the last are of at least five years duration.

1. —— *This patient had a diagnosis of ovarian cancer in November 1972. She had a pelvic mass measuring 8 cm, and was markedly anemic. She had had twenty linear accelerator treatments in 1972, but the tumor recurred and she had additional surgery in December 1973, with a diagnosis of cyst-adenocarcinoma. She had further recurrences in November 1974 and had extensive surgery with partial resection of the bladder, small bowel, and fistulous sigmoid colon tract. She continued her autogenous vaccine, dietary measures, and BCG. She received no chemotherapy and no further radiation. She made a complete recovery and remains well to date. This case illustrates that, although there was recurrence following radiation and repeated surgery, with our treatment the patient fully recovered and remains so to date. She did not receive chemotherapy and had no bone marrow impairment.*

2. —— *This is a case of a male with metastatic breast cancer. He came to the clinic November 6, 1978. On September*

21, 1978, he had been found to have a well-differentiated adenocarcinoma of the right breast with metastases to three regional
lymph nodes. He had had surgery, but he refused both chemotherapy and radiation. Male breast cancer shows a low rate of
survival, particularly when there is metastatic disease of the adjacent lymph nodes. But this patient has continued with our
immunological program. He is well and disease-free today, without having had any other therapy.

3. —— This case demonstrates that metastatic cancer of
the liver can return to normal. After exploratory surgery in May
1977—laparotomy and exploration of the transverse colon—she
was diagnosed as having metastatic, infiltrating, moderately well-
differentiated adenocarcinoma of the colon. A sigmoid resection
and closure of a transverse colostomy was done on May 25, 1977.
A liver scan in August 1977 showed a normal liver and spleen
but in the interim she developed cancer of the liver, and a liver
scan in October 1977 showed several poorly defined areas of increased activity. These were diagnosed as probably metastases from
the known cancer of the colon. The spleen was normal and there
was no activity in the bone marrow. The patient was admitted
to the clinic on November 2, 1977, and placed on all modalities
of nutrition, vitamins, minerals. Her C.E.A. on arrival was 3.6
ng/ml. She states that she has liver scans every six months. Our
records show scan reports as follows: a. May 1981: at least one
perfusion defect involving the upper portion of the left lobe—
suspicious for neoplastic disease. b. October 1981: perfusion defect
in the left lobe of the liver is not apparent on this study. c.
November 1982: no evidence of metastic disease in the liver. Since
May 1979 the C.E.A. has remained below 1.25 ng/ml. To date,
April 1983, the patient remains well and sees us about twice a
year for a checkup.

4. —— This female patient came to us in April 1977 with
a history of bladder cancer, which had been excised. She remained
well on the dietary and immunological program until March 1979,
when she had a recurrence following poor compliance with our

program. She cleared again after reinforcement of the program and was again clear in January 1980. With absence from the clinic for one year, she again recurred. She refused surgery at first but had the tumor removed. She started the program again and cleared again as of July 1982. Her own doctor urged this patient to have a radical cystectomy because of a poorly differentiated transitional cell tumor the previous March. At the time of surgery for the radical cystectomy, November 1982, no cancer was found, only dysplasia. This history shows conclusively that cancer of the bladder, even though recurrent, is treatable by dietary and immunological therapy.

5. —— *This is a case of lymphoma clearing without surgery, radiation, or chemotherapy. In September 1979 a biopsy revealed non-Hodgkins lymphoma. A lymphangiogram was done in October 1979 and reported at the University of New Mexico School of Medicine at Albuquerque. The test showed a large involved node in the midleft periaortic chain. Gallium scan showed increased uptake in that region in the left neck, and some patchy uptake in the liver plus an abdominal mass. No treatment was given. The disease was widespread but the patient felt good and was told he could live ten to fifteen years. The patient was admitted to our clinic, October 10, 1979, and put on the program. When his BCG was active a week later, he was allowed to return home while he remained on the program. He returned on December 26, 1979, to get another BCG and supplies. He stayed two days for treatment and then returned home. He returned again, March 31, 1980, for tests, revaccination with BCG, and supplies. December 1, 1980, ultrasound showed no other enlarged nodes but there was evidence of enlarged inguinal nodes. The patient returns now every four to six months for checkups and revaccination as well as to get supplies and ultrasound tests. Prognosis note of August 3, 1981, showed that he was completely free of any tumors, according to all objective and subjective tests, and he is back to work, driving a truck full time. His last visit to date was December 30, 1982, and he remains totally well by all tests and examinations.*

6. —— *This case shows that prostatic cancer can be controlled by dietary immunological procedures alone. A fifty-two-year-old male came to the clinic in July 1977 with a diagnosis of a well-differentiated adenocarcinoma of the prostate diagnosed by needle biopsy. The prostatic alkaline phosphatase was elevated. He had some difficulty with urinary flow. He had received small doses of DES daily. Symptoms included bloody semen on occasion and dysuria. No evidence of metastatic spread outside the capsule indentation base of the bladder. An echogenic area was found in the posterior area of the bladder. By 1979 the PAP was normal. There were no nodules in the prostate and the urinary stream was normal, although mild enlargement remained without symptoms. He has had the full program. PPD shows adequate reaction. He discontinued DES after the first year. Ultrasound shows no changes in past years.*

7. —— *This case illustrates that although the neoplastic state has existed for years and has been unsuccessfully treated by many modalities, it is still possible to redeem the situation and clear the patient of disease. This fifty-five-year-old female came to the clinic in May 1975. She had had a modified radical of the right breast in 1970. She had metastases to the right axilla and to the bone. She had several local recurrences removed surgically and then radiated. She had an oophorectomy in 1973. This removal helped for a while, but in 1974 she had a recurrent tumor removed from the right axilla. Adrenalectomy was recommended, but she refused. She then went to the Contreras Clinic in Tijuana, Mexico, with little result. When she came to us she had bone metastasis, general debility, and much pain. She did well in the interim but abandoned the program in the summer of 1982. More local nodes were removed and small nodes recurred again later in 1982. These were injected locally with antigen and cleared. Bone pain is gone. Chest wall is clear. She feels well.*

8. —— *This case illustrates that in selected cases simple lumpectomy is sufficient, in addition to the immunization program, in breast cancer. This seventy-seven-year-old female patient*

came to the clinic on February 8, 1977, with a lump in her left breast. It was 1.5 by 2 cm large and was located in the lower left inner quadrant. Mild dimpling of the skin and no discharge. She chose to be preimmunized prior to surgery with autogenous vaccine, BCG, and to start on a dietary program. She had no evidence of metastases. She had the surgical lumpectomy only and continued her dietary and immunization maintenance to the present time. She is disease-free.

9. —— *This patient was found to have a nodule in the left axilla in August 1973, during a routine physical examination. It was removed surgically and biopsy showed it to be a metastatic melanoma from an unknown site. The mass recurred. In September he had a radical axillary node dissection followed by radiation. He had many nevi over the body but the primary was never found. In the ensuing ten years, he has followed the entire therapeutic routine at the clinic. He has remained in excellent health continuing his preventive therapy. Because the original tumor was never found and because it recurred as metastatic disease, the combination of surgery, radiation, and immunotherapy has been most effective.*

10. —— *This case illustrates that discontinuance of tobacco and alcohol, good nutrition, large and frequent doses of vitamin C, immunizations with autogenous vaccine, and repeated BCGs have resulted in a complete remission at this time. This forty-four-year-old male came to the clinic on March 19, 1982. Two years previously he had had a resection plus a skin graft over his right lower back performed at the Stanford Clinic. Two recurrences necessitated a right axillary and right groin dissection. In spite of these measures, the melanoma recurred in three ribs. It was recommended that he have a rib resection. Following discontinuation of tobacco, a full vaccine and dietary program, plus frequent intravenous vitamin C, a recent CAT scan shows the ribs totally healed. In spite of repeated surgery and chemotherapy his lesions recurred and did not heal until he received immunotherapy supported by essential dietary factors.*

BIBLIOG-RAPHY

INDEX OF REPRINTS
OF VIRGINIA LIVINGSTON-WHEELER
(WUERTHELE-CASPE), M.D.

"Scleroderma treated with Promin—with report of a case," *The Journal of the Medical Society of New Jersey*, Vol. 44, p. 52, 1947.

"Etiology of Scleroderma—a preliminary clinical report," *The Journal of the Medical Society of New Jersey*, 1947.

"Microorganisms associated with Neoplasms," New York Microscopial Society Bulletin, No. 2., Vol. 2, New York, August 1948.

"Cultural Properties and Pathogenicity of Certain Microorganisms obtained from Various Proliferative and Neoplastic Diseases," *American Journal of the Medical Sciences*, 220, 638, December 1950.

"Microbiology of Cancer, Neoplastic Infection of Men and Animals," Atti Del VI Congresso Internazionale Di Microbiologia, Roma, Vol. 6, Sez. XVII, pg. 3–9, Sept. 1953.

"Some Aspects of the Microbiology of Cancer," *Journal of the American Medical Women's Association*," Vol. 8, No. 1, pg. 7–12, Jan. 1953.

"Neoplastic Infections of Man and Animals," *Journal of the American Medical Women's Association*, Vol. 10, No. 8, pg. 261–266, August 1955.

"Intracellular Acid-Fast Microorganism—Isolated from two cases of Hepato-lenticular Degeneration," *Journal of the American Medical Women's Association*, Vol. 11, No. 4, pg. 120–129, April 1956.

"Mycobacterial Forms in Myocardial Vascular Disease," *Journal of the American Medical Women's Association*, Vol. 20, No. 5, pp. 449–452, May 1965.

"An Experimental Biologic Approach to the Treatment of Neoplastic Disease," *Journal of the American Medical Women's Association,* Vol.20, No. 9, pg. 859–866, September 1965.

"A Specific Type of Organism Cultivated From Malignancy: Bacteriology and Proposed Classification," Annals of the New York Academy of Sciences, Vol. 174, Article 2, pg. 636–654, Oct. 1970.

"Toxic Fractions Obtained From Tumor Isolates And Related Clinical Implications," Annals of the New York Academy of Sciences, Vol. 174, Article 2, pg. 675–689, October 30, 1970.

"Demonstration of Progenitor Cryptocides in the Blood of Patients With Collagen and Neoplastic Diseases," N.Y. Academy of Sciences reprint. By Virginia Wuerthele-Caspe, Livingston, and Afton Munk Livingston USD. Submitted November 9, 1971; revision accepted Jan. 28, 1972

"Some Cultural, Immunological, and Biochemical Properties of Progenitor Cryptocides," Transactions of the New York Academy of Sciences, Series II, Vol. 36, No. 6, pg. 569–582, June 1974.

"The Role of Nutrition in the Immunotherapy of Cancer," *Journal of the International Academy of Preventive Medicine,* Vol. V, No. 2, 1981.

"Production of Choriogonadotropin in vitro by a Microbe, Progenitor Cryptocides, a member of the order Actinomycetales," V. Livingston-Wheeler, San Diego; O.W. Wheeler, San Diego; J.J. Majnarich, Seattle; 1982.

CONFIRMATORY PAPERS

Chicken Cancer in Relation to Humans

V. Ellerman and O. Bang. "Experimentelle Leukamie by Huhnern." *Zent. F. Bakteriologie,* 46, 595–609 (1908).

Dr. Peyton Rous. "A Transmissible Avian Neoplasm." *J. Experimental Medicine,* 12, 696–705 (1910).

Dr. Peyton Rous. "A Sarcoma of the Fowl Transmissible by an Agent Separable from the Tumor Cells." *J. Experimental Medicine,* 13, 397–410 (1911).

Dr. Peyton Rous and James B. Murphy. "The Nature of the Filterable Agent Causing a Sarcoma of the Fowl." *J. Am. Med. Assoc.* 58, 1938 (1912).

James B. Murphy and Peyton Rous. "The Behavior of Chicken Sarcoma Implanted in the Developing Embryo." *J. Experimental Medicine*, 15, 119–132 (1912).

Peyton Rous and James B. Murphy. "The Histological Signs of Resistance to a Transmissible Sarcoma of the Fowl." *J. Experimental Medicine*, 15, 270–286 (1912).

Dr. Elise L'Esperance. "Studies in Hodgkin's Disease." *Ann. Surg.*, 93:162–168 (1931).

Virginia Wuerthele-Caspe, Eleanor Alexander-Jackson, John A. Anderson, James Hillier, Roy M. Allen, and Lawrence W. Smith. "Cultural Properties and Pathogenicity of Certain Micro-organisms Obtained from Various Proliferative and Neoplastic Diseases." *Am. J. Med. Sci.* 220, 638–648 (1950).

Dr. Francisco Duran Reynals. "Neoplastic Infection and Cancer." *Am. J. Med.* N.Y. Vol. VIII, No. 4, 440–511 (1950).

Conversations with Dr. Peyton Rous, at Rockefeller Institute, New York City and at Rutgers Laboratory of Presbyterian Hospital, Newark, New Jersey, 1949–53.

Dr. Virginia Wuerthele-Caspe Livingston, M.D. "Neoplastic Infections of Man and Animals," *J. Am. Med. Women's Assoc.* 8, 1:7–12 (1953).

——. "Microbiology of Cancer, Neoplastic Infection in Man and Animals." *Atti del VI Congresso Internationale de Microbiologia, Roma*, Vol. 6, Sec. XVII, 3–9 (1953).

Virginia Wuerthele-Caspe, Eleanor Alexander-Jackson, and Lawrence Weld Smith. "Some Aspects of the Microbiology of Cancer." *J. Am. Medical Women's Assoc.* 8, 7–12 (1953).

Florence B. Siebert and L. F. Affronti. "Growth and Morphological Variability of Three Similar Strains of Intermittently Acid-fast Organisms Isolated from Mouse and Human Malignant Tissue." *Growth* 26, 181–208 (1962).

Virginia Wuerthele-Caspe Livingston and Eleanor Alexander-Jackson. "An Experimental Biological Approach to the Treatment of Neoplastic Disease." *J. Am. Med. Women's Assoc.* 20, 858–866 (1965).

Eleanor Alexander-Jackson. "Mycoplasma (PPLO) Isolated from Rous Sarcoma Virus," *Growth* 30, 199–228 (1966).

Dr. Virginia Wuerthele-Caspe Livingston, Eleanor Alexander-Jackson. "A Specific Type of Organism Cultivated from Malignancy Bacteriology and Proposed Classification." *Ann. N.Y. Academy Sci.* Vol. 174, 636–654 (1970). Oral pres. 1969.

"Chicken Cancer Called Widespread Enough to Pose 'Nightmares' for Poultry Industry." *Wall Street Journal*, February 10, 1970.

Eleanor Alexander-Jackson. "Ultraviolet Spectrogramic Studies of Rous Sarcoma Virus." *Ann. N.Y. Academy Sci.* Vol. 174, 765–781 (1970).

Dr. Virginia Wuethele-Caspe Livingston, M.D. *Cancer: A New Breakthrough.* San Diego: Livingston-Wheeler Foundation, pp. 107–115, 1972.

————. *The Microbiology of Cancer: A Compendium*. San Diego: Livingston-Wheeler Foundation, 1977.

Jack G. Makari. "Association between Marek's Herpesvirus and Human Cancer. I. Detection of Cross-reaching Antigens between Chicken Tumors and Human Tumors." *Oncology* 28, 164–176 (1973).

Jack. G. Makari. "Association between Marek's Herpesvirus and Human Cancer. II. Detection of Structural Viral Antigens in Chicken Tumors and Human Tumors." *Oncology* 28, 177–183 (1973).

Elizabeth McCullough. "Can Eggs be a Source of Cancer?" February 1, 1979. (Unpublished paper; copies available at Livingston-Wheeler Clinic, San Diego.)

Drs. Virginia Livingston-Wheeler and Owen Webster Wheeler. *Conquest of Cancer Transcripts*, edited by Carolyn Collins. San Diego: Livingston-Wheeler Foundation (1983).

Dr. Alsoph Corwin. Introduction to *Conquest of Cancer Transcripts*, Livingston-Wheeler Clinic and Foundation, ed. Carolyn Collins, San Diego, 1983.

Pathology

Lawrence W. Smith, "Pathologic Changes Induced in Animals by Microorganisms Recovered from Cases of Human Cancer," from the Bureau of Biological Research for the Study of Proliferative Diseases—Rutgers University Branch at Presbyterian Hospital, Newark, N.J.

Oncology and the Retinoids

"Nutrition, the Changing Scene," *The Lancet*, April 16, 1983; from W. Bollag, *Vitamin A and Retinoids: From Nutrition to Pharmacotherapy in Dermatology and Oncology*.

Scleroderma

N. Delmotte and L. van der Meiren, "Recherches bactériologiques concernant la sclérodermie," in *Dermatologica*.

Dermatologische Zeitschrift-Separatum, Vol. 107, No. 3, 1953.

Alan R. Cantwell, Jr., M.D., and Dan W. Kelso, "Acid-Fast Bacteria in Scleroderma and Morphea," reprinted from the *Archives of Dermatology*, Vol. 4, American Medical Association, June 1941.

Production of Choriogonadotropin by P. Cryptocides

Herman Cohen and Alice Strampp, "Bacterial Synthesis of Substance Similar to Human Chorionic Gonadotropin," in Proceedings of the Society for Experimental Biology and Medicine, Academic Press, Vol. 152, No. 3, July 1976.

John A. Kellen, M.D., Ph.D., Arnost Kolin, M.D., and Hernan F. Acevedo, Ph.D., "Effects of Antibodies to Choriogonadotropin in Malignant Growth, I. Rat 3230 AC Mammary Adenocarcinoma," *Cancer*, reprinted, Vol. 49, No 11, June 1, 1982

John A. Kellen, M.D., Ph.D., Arnost Kolin, M.D., Apkar Mirakian, and Hernan F. Acevedo, Ph.D., "Effects of Antibodies to Choriogonadotropin in Malignant Growth, II. Solid Transplantable Rat Tumors," *Cancer Immunology and Immunotherapy*, Springer-Verlag, 1982.

Index of Papers by Dr. Irene Corey Diller

"Tumor Incidence in ICR/Albino and C57/B16JNIcr Male Mice Injected Organisms Cultured from Mouse Malignant Tissues," Institute for Cancer Research, Philadelphia, Pa., in *Growth*, pg. 38, 507–517, 1974.

"Experiments with Mammalian Tumor Isolates," Annals of the New York Academy of Sciences, Vol. 174, Art. 2, pg. 655–675, 1970.

"Three Similar Strains of Pleomorphic Acid-Fast Organisms Isolated From Rat and Mouse Tissues and From Human Blood," *American Review of Respiratory Diseases*, Vol. 86, No. 6, Dec. 1962.

"Intracellular Acid-Fast Organisms Isolated from Malignant Tissues," Transactions of the American Microscopial Society, 84 (1) pg. 138–148, 1965.

"Growth and Morphological Variability of Three Similar Strains of Intermittently Acid-Fast Organisms Isolated from Mouse and Human Malignant Tissues," in *Growth*, 26, pg. 181–208, 1962.

Abstracts of Papers Demonstrating the Microbial Origin of Cancer. Translated and Collected by Irene Corey Diller, Ph. D.

Crofton, W. M., "Therapeutic Immunization."

Fonti, Clara, "Etiopatogenese del Cancro." Inst. Editoriale Cisalpino A. Nicola & C. Milano-Varese, 273 pp. 27 p. bibl. 1958.

Gerlach, Franz, "Krebs und obligater Pilzparasitismus." Urban u. Schwarzenburg, Wien, 211, p. 115 pl. 1948.

Glover, T. J. "The Bacteriology of Cancer," *Canada Lancet and Practitioner* 74: 1–19, 1930.

Inoue, Sakae and Marcus Singer, *Nature*, Vol. 205, Jan. 23, 1965.

Mazet, Georges, "Étude bactériologique sur le maladie d'Hodgkin." Extrait de Montpellier Medicalle, Juillet-Aout, 1941.

Mori, Nello, "Virus filtrabili e cancro secondo la mia ipotesi (1914) della loro natura micetica." *Pregresso Medico* 6:3-31, 1950.

A proposito della mia concezione etiopatogenetica simbioparassitaria inframicetica del cancro. Atti Congresso Nazionale della Legge Italiana per la lotta contro i tumori. p. 259–268, June 1953.

Scott, M. J. "Use of antiserum for Treatment of Cancer."

Seibert, Florence B., et al. "Isolation of pleomorphic organisms from cancer."

Von Brehmer, Wilhelm, *Siphonospora polymorpha*, Wien, Linck-Verlag, 1947.

Villequez, E. *La parasitisme latent des cellules du sang chez l'homme, en particulier le sang du cancereux.* Librerie Maloine, Paris, 1955.

Papers by Dr. Eleanor Alexander-Jackson

"Ultraviolet Spectrogramic Microscope Studies of Rous Sarcoma Virus Cultured in Cell-free Medium," Annals of the New York Academy of Sciences, Vol. 174, Art. 2, pg. 765–781, 1970.

"Mycoplasma (PPLO) Isolated From Rous Sarcoma Virus," *Growth*, 30, pg. 199–228, 1966.

"Lesions Developing After Inoculation of Newborn Rats with a Pleomorphic Organism Isolated from a Leprosy Patient," paper presented by invitation at the First Interamerican Congress of Experimental Leprology, Buenos Aires, June, 1961.

Suggested Reading of Important Papers and Books

Acevedo, Hernan F. et al. "Human Chorionic Gonadotropin in Cancer Cells I. Identification in *in vivo* and *in vitro* Cancer Cell Systems," in Press: Proc. Third Intern. Symp. Detec. Prev. Cancer; Editor: H. E. Nieburgs, Marcel Dekker, Inc. New York, New York, 1976.

Addicott, Fredrick T., Jessye Lorene Lyon. "Physiology of Abscisic Acid and Related Substances." *Annual Review of Plant Physiology.* Vol. 20, 1969.

Baldwin, R. W., et al. (eds.) *Cancer Immunology and Immunotherapy*, Vol. 1, Nos. 1/2, 1976.

Baltimore, David. "Viruses, Polymerases, and Cancer," *Science*, Vol. 192, May 14, 1976.

Bansal, S. C., and H. O. Sjogren. "'Unblocking' Serum Activity *in vitro* in the Polyoma System may Correlate with Antitumor Effects of Antiserum *in vivo*," in Letters to Nature, *Nature New Biology*, Vol. 233, September 15, 1971.

Berard, Costan W. (Moderator NIH Conference). "Current Concepts of Leukemia and Lymphoma: Etiology, Pathogenesis, and Therapy." *Annals of Internal Medicine* 85:351–366, 1976.

Berger, Patricia J. et al. "Phenolic Plant Compounds Functioning as Reproductive Inhibitors in *Microtus montanus*." *Science*, Vol. 195, February 11, 1977.

Bissell, Mina J. et al. "Preferential Inhibition at the Growth of Virus-Transformed Cells in Culture by Rifazone 8_2, a New Rifamucin Derivative." Proc. Nat. Acad. Sci. USA, Vol. 71, No. 6, pp. 2520–2524, June 1974.

Brennan, Richard O. *Coronary? Cancer? God's Answer: Prevent It!* (Harvest House, 1979).

Bryan, William T. K. and Marian P. Bryan. "Cytotoxic Reactions—How they can be used as a new Immunologic Test" (Paper).

Cameron, Ewan, and Linus Pauling. "Supplemental ascorbate in the supportive treatment of cancer: Prolongation of survival times in terminal human cancer." Proc. Nat. Acad. Sci. USA, Vol. 73, No. 10, pp. 3685–3689, October 1976.

Cancer Chemotherapy, Year Book Medical Publishers Inc., Chicago, 1975.

Diller, Irene Corey, et al. "The Effect of Aqueous Spleen Extract on Growth of Tumor Cells in Mice." *Growth*, Vol. XIII, pp. 27–44, Paper No. 349, 1949.

Dulbecco, Renato. "From the Molecular Biology of Oncogenic DNA Viruses to Cancer." *Science*, Vol. 192, April 30, 1976.

Duran-Reynals, F. "Neoplastic Infection and Cancer." *The American Journal of Medicine*, N.Y. Vol. VIII, No. 4, pp. 490–511, April 1950.

Ghosh, Nimai K., and Rody P. Cox. "Production of human chorionic gonadotropin in HeLa cell cultures." *Nature*, Vol. 259, No. 5542, pp. 416–417, February 5, 1976.

Glasser, Robert J. *The Body Is the Hero.* (Random House, 1976).

Hersh, Evan, et al. "Host Defense, Chemical Immunosuppression, and the

Transplant Recipient. Relative Effects of Intermittent Versus Continuous Immunosuppressive Therapy with Reference to the Objectives of Treatment." *Transplantation Proceedings*, Vol. V, No. 3, September 1973.

Hersh, Evan M., et al. "BCG Vaccine and Its Derivatives—Potential, Practical Considerations, and Precautions in Human Cancer Immunotherapy." *JAMA*, Vol. 235, No. 6, February 9, 1976.

Holland, James F., and Emil Frei, III. *Cancer Medicine*, Lea & Febiger, 1974.

Holmes, E. Carmack, et al. "Immunotherapy of Cancer." *The Western Journal of Medicine*, 126:102–109, February 1977.

Jablonska, Stefanie. *Scleroderma and pseudoscleroderma*, Polish Medical Publishers, Warsaw, 1975.

Kufe, D. et al. "Burkitt's Tumors Contain Particles Encapsulating RNA-Instructed DNA Polymerase and High Molecular Weight Virus-Related RNA." Proc. Nat. Acad. Sci. USA, Vol. 70, No. 3, pp. 737–741, March 1973.

Kufe, D. W. et al. "Unique Nuclear DNA Sequences in the Involved Tissues of Hodgkin's and Burkitt's Lymphomas." Proc. Nat. Acad. Sci. USA, vol. 70, No. 12, Part II, pp. 3810–3814, Dec. 1973.

LeVeen, Harry H. et al. "Tumor Eradication by Radiofrequency Therapy. Response in 21 Patients." *JAMA*, Vol. 235, No. 20, May 17, 1976.

Makari, J. G. "Association between Marek's Herpesvirus and Human Cancer. II. Detection of Structural Viral Antigens in Chicken Tumors and Human Tumors." *Oncology*, 28:177–183, 1973.

Mankiewicz, E. "Antigenic Components shared by Bacteriophages and Phage-Hosts: Mycobacteria, Corynebacteria and Hela Cells." *Growth*, 29:125–139, 1965.

Marmor, Jane B. et al. "Tumor Cure and Cell Survival After Localized Radiofrequency Heating." Paper submitted to Cancer Research.

Marin, F. et al. "The Specificity of Carcino-Foetal Antigens of the Human Digestive Tract Tumors." *Europ. J. Cancer*, Vol. 8, pp. 315–321, Pergamon Press, 1972.

Mavligit, Gloria M. et al. "Prolongation of Postoperative Disease-Free Interval and Survival in Human Colorectal Cancer by B.C.G. or B.C.G. plus 5-Fluorouracil." *The Lancet*, Saturday, April 24, 1976.

Myers, John A. "Metabolic Aspects of Cancer," *Journal of Applied Nutrition*, Spring, 1976.

Naughton, Michael A. et al. "Localization of the B Chain of Human Chorionic Gonadotropin on Human Tumor Cells and Placental Cells." *Cancer Research* 35, 1887, 1890, July 1975.

Nauts, Helen C. "Beneficial Effects of Immunotherapy (Bacterial Toxins) on Sarcoma of the Soft Tissues, Other than Lymphosarcoma." Monograph

No. 16, Cancer Research Institute Inc. New York, 1975.

Peters, W. P. et al. "Biological and Biochemical Evidence for an Interaction Between Marek's Disease Herpesvirus and Avian Leukosis Virus *in vivo*." Proc. Nat. Acad. Sci. USA, Vol. 70, No. 11, pp. 3175–3178, November 1973.

Rojas, A. F. et al. "Levamisole in Advanced Human Breast Cancer." *The Lancet*, 31 January 1976.

Rosenthal, Sol Roy, et al. *BCG Vaccination and Leukemia Mortality*. Littleton, MA: Wright-PSG, 1980.

Schrauzer, Gerhard N. "Cancer Mortality Correlation Studies. II. Regional Associations of Mortalities with the Consumptions of Foods and other Commodities." *Medical Hypothesis* Vol. 2, March-April 1976.

Seibert, Florence B. "A Theory of Immunity in Tuberculosis." *Perspectives in Biology and Medicine*, Vol. III, No. 2, Winter 1960.

Seibert, Florence B. et al. "Decrease in spontaneous tumors by vaccinating C3H Mice with an homologous bacterial vaccine." IRCS International Research Communications System, March 1973.

Shamberger, R. J. et al. "Antioxidants and Cancer. I. Selenium in the Blood of Normals and Cancer Patients." *Journal of the National Cancer Institute*, 50(4): 863–870, 1973.

Shils, Maurice, E. "Nutrition and Cancer: Dietary Deficiency and Modifications." Cancer Epidemiology and Prevention—Current Concepts—American Lecture Series.

Sinkovics, Joseph G. "Progress in Clinical Immunotherapy for Tumors." *Postgraduate Medicine*, Vol. 59, No. 2, Feb. 1976.

Sporn, Michael B. et al. "Prevention of chemical carcinogenesis by vitamin A and its synthetic analogs (retinoids)." Nutrition and Cancer, Federation Proceedings, Vol. 35, No. 6, May 1, 1976.

Sporn, Michael B. "13-cis-Retinoic Acid: Inhibition of Bladder Carcinogenesis in the Rat." *Science*, Vol. 195, Feb. 4, 1977.

Suss, R., V. Kinzel, and J. D. Scribner. *Cancer Experiments and Concepts*. Springer-Verlag, New York, Heidelberg, Berlin, 1973.

Teasdale, F., et al. "Human Chorionic Gonadotropin: Inhibitory Effect on Mixed Lymphocyte Cultures." *Genec. Invest.* 4: 263–269, 1973.

Thomas, Lewis, *The Lives of a Cell*. New York: Viking, 1974.

Weinberg, Eugene D. "Iron and Susceptibility to Infectious Disease." *Science*, Vol. 184, May 31, 1974.

INDEX